Evidence-Based Public Health

Evidence-Based Public Health

ROSS C. BROWNSON
ELIZABETH A. BAKER
TERRY L. LEET
KATHLEEN N. GILLESPIE

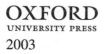

OXFORD
UNIVERSITY PRESS
2003

OXFORD
UNIVERSITY PRESS

Oxford   New York
Auckland   Bangkok   Buenos Aires   Cape Town   Chennai
Dar es Salaam   Delhi   Hong Kong   Istanbul   Karachi   Kolkata
Kuala Lumpur   Madrid   Melbourne   Mexico City   Mumbai   Nairobi
São Paulo   Shanghai   Singapore   Taipei   Tokyo   Toronto

Copyright © 2003 by Oxford University Press, Inc.

Published by Oxford University Press, Inc.
198 Madison Avenue, New York, New York 10016
http://www.oup.com

Oxford is a registered trademark of Oxford University Press

Library of Congress Cataloging-in-Publication Data
Evidence-based public health / Ross C. Brownson . . . [et al.].
p. ; cm.
Includes bibliographical references and index.
ISBN 0-19-514376-0 (acid-free paper)
1. Public health.   2. Evidence-based medicine.   I. Title: Evidence based public health.
II. Brownson, Ross C.
RA427 .E954 2003
362.1—dc21   2002018840

9 8 7 6 5 4 3 2 1

Printed in the United States of America
on acid-free paper

Foreword

When we hear the word *evidence*, most of us conjure up the mental picture of a courtroom, with opposing lawyers presenting their evidence, or of law enforcement personnel sifting through a crime scene for evidence to be used in judicial proceedings.

Evidence, so central to our notion of justice, is equally central to public health. This is because it should inform all of our judgments about what interventions to implement, in what populations, when, and how to determine both positive and sometimes negative effects of those interventions.

In public health there are four principal user groups for evidence.

Public health practitioners with executive and managerial responsibilities want to know what is the evidence for alternative strategies, be they policies, programs, or other activities. Too infrequently, busy practitioners find the time to ask the fundamental question, "What are the most important things I can do to improve the public's health?" In pursuit of answers, population-based data is the first prerequisite, covering health status, health risks, and health problems for the overall population and demographic subsegments. Also important are the population's attitudes and beliefs about various major health problems. The second prerequisite is data on potential interventions. What are they? What do we know about each? What is their individual and conjoint effectiveness in improving health in the populations we are serving? This marriage of information can lead to a rational prioritization of opportunities, constrained only by resources and feasibility.

More often, public health practitioners have a more narrow set of options. Funds from federal, state, or local governments are earmarked for a specific purpose, such as surveillance and treatment of sexually transmitted diseases, inspection of retail food establishments, or treatment for substance abusers. Still, the practitioner has the opportunity, even the obligation, to survey the evidence carefully for alternative ways to achieve the desired health goals. Those on the front lines share the responsibility of seeking evidence on how they can be most effective and efficient.

The next user group includes policy makers at local, regional, state, national, and international levels. They are faced with macrolevel decisions on how to allocate the public resources for which they have been elected stewards. This group has the additional responsibility of making policies on controversial public issues. Under what conditions should gun ownership be allowed? How much tax should be levied on cigarettes, and how should these tax revenues be used? Should needle exchange programs be legal for intravenous drug addicts? Should treatment be the required alternative for perpetrators of nonviolent offenses who committed crimes while abusing alcohol or other drugs? Good politicians want to know the evidence for the effects of options they are being asked to consider or may want to propose.

Key stakeholders are a third user group for evidence. This group includes the public, especially those who vote, as well as interest groups formed to support or oppose specific policies, such as the legality of abortion, whether the community water supply should be fluoridated, or whether adults must be issued handgun licenses if they pass background checks. While ideology fuels passion on these issues, evidence can temper views or suggest a feasible range for compromise among opposing views. Sometimes voters are asked to weigh in on proposed policies, such as clean indoor air ordinances or bonds to support the emergency medical response system.

The final user group is composed of researchers on population health issues, who evaluate the impact of specific policies or programs. They both develop and use evidence to explore research hypotheses. Some of this group are primarily interested in the methods used to determine the quality and implications of research on population-based interventions. They frequently ask, "Was the study design appropriate?" and "What are the criteria for determining the adequacy of the study methods?"

This volume should be sweet music to each of these groups. Anyone needing to be convinced of the benefit of systematic development and synthesis of evidence for various public health purposes will quickly be won over. A step-by-step approach to compiling and assessing evidence of what works and what doesn't is well explicated. In a logical sequence, the reader is guided in how to use the results of his or her search for evidence in developing program or policy options, including the weighing of benefits versus barriers, and then in developing an action plan. To complete the cycle of science, the book describes how to evaluate whatever action is taken. Using this volume does not require extensive formal training in the key disciplines of epidemiology, biostatistics, or behavioral science, but those with strong disciplinary skills will also find much to learn from and put to practical use here.

If every public health practitioner absorbed and applied the key lessons in this volume, public health would enjoy a higher health return on the taxpayer's investment, and public health practitioners would be more successful in competing for limited public dollars because they would have evidence easy to support and difficult to refute. The same cannot be said for most of the competing requests for scarce public resources.

Jonathan E. Fielding, M.D., M.P.H., M.B.A.
Director of Public Health and Health Officer
County of Los Angeles
Professor of Health Services and Pediatrics
School of Public Health
University of California, Los Angeles

Preface

How much of our work in public health is evidence-based? Although the precise answer to that question cannot be known, it is almost certainly "Not enough!" Public health has successfully addressed many challenges, yet nearly every success story is a two-edged sword. Programs and policies have been implemented and, in some cases, positive results have been reported. Are there ways to take the lessons learned and apply them to other issues and settings? Here are a few examples:

- Over the past century, it has become clear that primary care physicians are in a position not only to treat disease but also to provide screening tests and counseling that will help prevent many diseases. Despite new evidence-based guidelines for clinical preventive services, many patients are not receiving scientifically proven interventions.
- The eradication of smallpox in 1980 demonstrated the powerful combination of vaccination, patient and worker education, and public health surveillance in disease reduction. Other vaccine-preventable diseases such as measles, hepatitis B, and rubella might also be eradicated with a global commitment.
- State-based programs to reduce tobacco use have demonstrated progress in California, Massachusetts, Florida, and elsewhere, yet many states and communities are not implementing comprehensive, evidence-based interventions to control tobacco use.
- Obesity is on a sharp rise among children in several countries. While we must focus on healthy eating and increasing activity, it remains unclear which interventions will be most effective in preventing obesity among children.
- There are large health disparities (e.g., among racial/ethnic groups, across so-

cioeconomic gradients) in the United States and many other countries. Although some promising behavioral interventions have been shown to address these disparities, new approaches are needed that include a focus on the "upstream" causes, such as income inequality, poor housing, racism, and lack of social cohesion.

As noted over a decade ago by the Institute of Medicine,[1] there are multiple reasons for the inefficiency and ineffectiveness of many public health efforts. There are at least three ways in which a public health program or policy may not reach stated goals for success:

1. Choosing an intervention approach whose effectiveness is not established in the scientific literature
2. Selecting a potentially effective program or policy yet achieving only weak, incomplete implementation or "reach," thereby failing to attain objectives
3. Conducting an inadequate or incorrect evaluation that results in a lack of generalizable knowledge on the effectiveness of a program or policy

To enhance evidence-based practice, this book addresses all three possibilities and attempts to provide practical guidance on how to choose, carry out, and evaluate evidence-based programs and policies in public health settings. It also begins to address a fourth, overarching need for a highly trained public health workforce. Our book deals not only with *finding* and *using* scientific evidence, but also with implementation and evaluation of interventions that *generate* new evidence on effectiveness. Because all these topics are broad and require multidisciplinary skills and perspectives, each chapter covers the basic issues and provides multiple examples to illustrate important concepts. In addition, each chapter provides linkages to diverse literature and selected websites for readers wanting more detailed information. Readers should note that websites are volatile, and when a link changes, a generic search engine may be useful in locating the new Web address.

We began to see a need for this book through our experiences in public health practice, health care delivery, and teaching. Much of the book's new material originated from several courses that we have taught over the past four years. One that we offer with the Missouri Department of Health and Senior Services, "Evidence-Based Decision-Making in Public Health," is designed for midlevel managers in state health agencies and leaders of city and county health agencies. We developed a national version of this course with the Association of State and Territorial Chronic Disease Program Directors and the Centers for Disease Control and Prevention. The same course has also been adapted for use in Illinois, West Virginia, Austria, and Russia.

The format for our book is very similar to the approach taken in the course.

Chapter 1 provides the rationale for evidence-based approaches to decision making in public health. Chapter 2 presents concepts of causality that help in determining when scientific evidence is sufficient for public health action. Chapter 3 describes a set of analytic tools that can be extremely useful in finding and evaluating evidence—these include economic evaluation, public health surveillance, meta-analysis, and expert guidelines. The remaining six chapters lay out a sequential framework for

1. Developing an initial statement of the issue
2. Quantifying the issue
3. Searching the scientific literature and organizing information
4. Developing and prioritizing program options
5. Developing an action plan and implementing interventions
6. Evaluating the program or policy

While an evidence-based process is not linear, these six steps are described in some detail to illustrate their importance in making scientifically based decisions about public health programs and policies.

This book has been written for public health professionals without extensive formal training in the public health sciences (behavioral science, biostatistics, environmental and occupational health, epidemiology, public health administration) and for students in public health and preventive medicine. We hope the book will be useful for state and local health agencies, nonprofit organizations, academic institutions, health care organizations, and national public health agencies. Although it is intended primarily for a North American audience, examples are drawn from many parts of the world, and we believe that the key principles and skills are applicable in both developed and developing countries. The future of public health holds enormous potential, and public health professionals have more tools at their fingertips than ever before to meet these challenges. We hope this book will be a useful resource for bridging research and the practice of public health.

R. C. B.
E. A. B.
T. L. L.
K. N. G.

REFERENCE

1. IOM. Committee for the Study of the Future of Public Health. *The Future of Public Health*. Washington, DC: National Academy Press, 1988.

Acknowledgments

We are grateful to numerous individuals who contributed to the development of this book and reviewed earlier drafts of chapters.

We particularly wish to thank Garland Land, who chaired the original work group that developed the concept for our course, "Evidence-Based Decision Making in Public Health." Laura Caisley produced the first draft of this book's glossary and coordinated our course logistics. Carolyn Harris also coordinated the course until May 2001. Our national advisory group for the course included Chris Maylahn, Donna Nichols, Margret O'Neall, Deborah Porterfield, Shah Roohi, Paul Siegel, and Carol Stanwyck. We have received support from the Centers for Disease Control and Prevention and the Chronic Disease Directors. We are especially grateful to Gary Hogelin and Paul Siegel.

Chapter reviewers included the following individuals: Barb Arrington, Suzanne Bakdash, Bill Baldyga, Peter Briss, Carol Brownson, Claudia Campbell, Simon Chapman, Jonathan Fielding, Judith Garrard, Jim Gurney, Anne Korr, Marshall Kreuter, Brick Lancaster, Garland Land, Gene Lengerich, Chris Maylahn, Joanne Mitten, David Nelson, Margret O'Neall, Edith Parker, Pat Remington, Paul Siegel, Tom Sims, Eduardo Simoes, Steve Teutsch, Robert Thompson, Fred Wolinsky, and Stephanie Zaza. Sue Foerster and Jim Romeis contributed information for two chapters.

Finally, we are indebted to Jeff House, Oxford University Press, who provided valuable advice and ideas throughout the production of this book.

Contents

Evidence-Based Public Health

1

The Need for Evidence-Based Public Health

> If we did not respect the evidence, we would have very little
> leverage in our quest for the truth.
>
> —Carl Sagan

The many accomplishments of modern public health can be lauded, including
the thirty-year gain in life expectancy in the United States in the twentieth
century.[1] Much of this increase can be attributed to the provision of safe water
and food, sewage treatment and disposal, tobacco use prevention, injury prevention, control of infectious diseases through immunization, and other
population-based, public health interventions.[2] Despite these successes, many
additional public health challenges remain. To meet expectations for continuing
improvement (e.g., achieving *Healthy People 2010* goals[3]), a drive toward more
widespread use of evidence-based strategies for effectively addressing current
challenges in public health is needed.

Ideally, public health practitioners always incorporate scientific evidence in
making management decisions, developing policies, and implementing programs. In reality, however, these decisions are often based on short-term demands rather than long-term study, and policies and programs are sometimes
developed around anecdotal evidence. These concerns were noted over a decade
ago when the Institute of Medicine determined that decision making in public
health is often driven by "crises, hot issues, and concerns of organized interest
groups." (p. 4).[4] To address these issues in a more evidence-based approach to
decision making often requires enhanced individual skills, wider use of data and
analytic tools, and a more favorable organizational climate. At the organizational
level, it has been suggested that there is sparse scientific evidence to guide
decisions about how to develop, operate, or even determine what constitutes an
effective health department.[5]

This chapter includes four major sections: (1) relevant background issues,

including an overview of evidence-based medicine and other concepts underlying evidence-based public health; (2) several key characteristics of an
evidenced-based process; (3) a brief sketch of a framework for evidence-based
decision making in public health practice; and (4) a summary of barriers and
opportunities for widespread implementation of evidence-based approaches. A
major goal of this introductory chapter is to move the process of decision making
toward a proactive approach that incorporates effective use of scientific evidence
and data. Macrolevel issues that determine whether an entire public health system is effective are beyond the book's scope. The literature at that level is
developing and covers issues such as performance monitoring, fiscal accountability, and workforce development.[5]

BACKGROUND

As a backdrop, it is useful to present key definitions, the basic tenets of evidence-
based medicine, and several issues that are important to consider when attempting to make the practice of public health more evidence based.

Key Definitions

At the most basic level, evidence involves "the available body of facts or information indicating whether a belief or proposition is true or valid."[6] For a public
health professional, these "facts" are often data—including epidemiologic (quantitative) data, results of program or policy evaluations, and qualitative data—for
use in decision making and priority setting. Jenicek has defined evidence-based
practice as the "use of epidemiological insight while studying and applying
research, clinical, and public health experience and findings in clinical practice,
health programs, and health policies."[7]

The definition of evidence-based public health has been broadened to include
"the development, implementation, and evaluation of effective programs and
policies in public health through application of principles of scientific reasoning,
including systematic uses of data and information systems, and appropriate use
of behavioral science theory and program planning models."[8] From such an
approach, activities in public health practice are explicitly linked with the underlying scientific evidence that demonstrates effectiveness.

Evidence-based public health involves the development and implementation
of effective programs and policies. A public health program can be defined as
a structured intervention with the intent of improving the health of the total
population or a subpopulation at particularly high risk. Health policies are "those
laws, regulations, formal and informal rules and understandings that are adopted

on a collective basis to guide individual and collective behavior."[9] Policy interventions are actions that alter or control the legal, social, economic, and physical environment[10] and are supported by the notion that individuals are strongly influenced by the sociopolitical and cultural environment in which they act.

Evolution of Evidence-Based Medicine

The concept of evidence-based medicine has grown in prominence in recent years.[11–14] It involves the delivery of optimal individual patient care through integration of current best evidence on pathophysiological knowledge and patient preferences. A simplified flowchart depicting evidence-based medicine is shown in Figure 1–1. Key skills include the ability to track down, critically appraise, and rapidly incorporate scientific evidence into a clinician's practice. Clinical evidence is weighted in three areas: validity, importance, and applicability to patients of particular interest.[7] Sackett and Rosenberg have described five essential steps in the practice of evidence-based medicine:[15]

1. Convert information needs into answerable questions
2. Track down, with maximum efficiency, the best evidence with which to answer them (from the clinical examination, the diagnostic laboratory, the published literature, or other sources)
3. Critically appraise that evidence performance for its validity (closeness to the truth) and usefulness (clinical applicability)

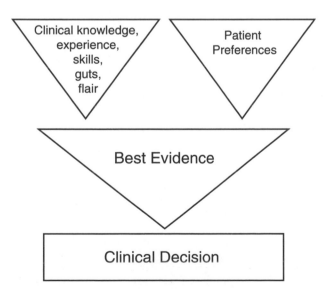

FIGURE 1–1. Flowchart of evidence-based medicine (adapted from Jenicek[7]).

4. Apply the results of this appraisal in clinical practice
5. Evaluate performance

An additional step may involve the teaching of evidence-based skills to clinicians.[16] Among the obstacles to increasing use of evidence-based medicine among clinicians are inadequate resources and skills, limited time, lack of physician "buy-in," the perception of a cookbook approach, and inadequate information systems.[17] Principles of evidence-based medicine have also been applied in a variety of medical subspecialties, nursing, dentistry, and clinical nutrition. In addition, new journals, including *ACP Journal Club, Evidence-Based Medicine*, have been launched that attempt to enhance the uses of evidence in clinical practice.

Evidence-based approaches are embodied in clinical guidelines, defined as "systematically developed statements to assist practitioner and patient decisions about appropriate health care for specific clinical circumstances."[18] Clinical guidelines have been especially important in preventive medicine, where they influence decisions at the level of individual clinicians as well as in helping to inform effective health policies.[19] As clinical guidelines have evolved, three important points have emerged:[20] 1) a systematic review of the evidence should be at the heart of every guideline; 2) the group assembled to translate the evidence into a guideline should be multidisciplinary; and 3) the development of guidelines requires sufficient resources (both in terms of people and financial support). Clinical and community guidelines are described in Chapter 3.

Differences between Evidence-Based Approaches in Medicine and Public Health. There are important distinctions between evidence-based approaches in medicine and in public health (Table 1–1). First, the quality and volume of evidence differ. Medical studies of pharmaceuticals and procedures often rely on randomized controlled trials of individuals, the most scientifically rigorous

Table 1–1. Key Differences between Evidence-Based Medicine and Evidence-Based Public Health

Characteristic	Evidence-Based Medicine	Evidence-Based Public Health
Quality of evidence	Experimental studies	Observational and quasi-experimental studies
Volume of evidence	Larger	Smaller
Time from intervention to outcome	Shorter	Longer
Professional training	More formal, with certification and/or licensing	Less formal, no standard certification
Decision making	Individual	Team

of epidemiologic studies. In contrast, public health interventions are likely to rely on cross-sectional studies, quasi-experimental designs, and time-series analyses. These studies sometimes lack a comparison group, which may limit the quality of the evidence for some interventions. Over the past fifty years, there have been approximately one million randomized controlled trials of medical treatments.[14] Even with this large number of trials, effectiveness is not proven for most of what is done in medicine.[19] There are many fewer studies of the effectiveness of public health interventions. Population-based studies often have a longer time period between intervention and outcome. An intervention to reduce smoking may have the ultimate outcome of reducing lung cancer deaths, yet it would take decades to evaluate this long-term endpoint. The formal training of persons working in public health is much more variable than in medicine. Unlike medicine, public health relies on a variety of disciplines, and there is not a single (or even small number of) academic credential(s) that "certifies" a public health practitioner. In the United States, for example, fewer than half of the 500,000 individuals in the public health workforce have had formal training in a public health discipline such as epidemiology or health education.[21] An even smaller percentage of these professionals have formal graduate training from a school of public health or other public health program. And finally, a decision in medicine often is made by a single physician, whereas public health decisions are usually made by teams with many varied points of view.

Other Underpinnings of Evidence-Based Public Health

As you begin to apply methods for making public health more evidence based, it is useful to consider the types of evidence available, their common characteristics, and their scope and quality.

Types of Evidence. Two types of evidence can be distinguished (Table 1–2). The first involves analytic data on the importance of a particular health condition and its link with some preventable risk factor. For example, a large body

Table 1–2. Comparison of the Types of Scientific Evidence

Characteristic	Type I	Type II
Typical data/relationship	Strength of preventable risk–disease relationship	Relative effectiveness of public health intervention
Common setting	Clinic or controlled community setting	Socially intact groups or community-wide
Quantity of evidence	More	Less
Action	"Something should be done."	"This should be done."

Table 1–3. Selected Examples of Prevention Effectiveness for Type I Evidence

Prevention Type[a]	Undesired Outcome	Annual U.S. Incidence without Prevention Measure	Prevention Method	Effectiveness (%)	Economic Analysis	Persons at Risk Covered by Method (%)
Primary	Measles	4,000,000	Vaccination	95–98	$16.85 per case prevented	By age 2, 50%–80%; by age 6, 98%
Secondary	Breast cancer deaths	50,000	Mammography screening of women >40 years	20–70	$45,000–$165,000 per year of life saved	15%–38%
Tertiary	Blindness from diabetes	24,000	Retinal screening, treatment	50	$100 per year of vision saved	60%–80%

[a]Primary prevention is directed at susceptible persons before they develop a particular disease (risk factor reduction); secondary prevention is directed to persons who are asymptomatic but who have developed biologic changes (early detection and treatment); tertiary prevention is directed at preventing disability in persons who have symptomatic disease (prevent complications and rehabilitation).

Source: Thacker et al.[22]

of research shows that the burden of childhood illness and death can be significantly reduced through widespread immunization. Factors important to consider include the condition's magnitude (number, incidence, or prevalence), severity (morbidity, mortality, disability), and preventability (what can be done to prevent the health condition). This type of evidence may lead one to the conclusion that *"something should be done"* (Type I Evidence). In many cases, the prevention measure can be quantified in terms of cases or deaths averted, effectiveness, and economic impact (Table 1–3).[22] The second type of evidence focuses on the relative effectiveness of specific interventions to address a particular health condition. In relation to immunization, for example, which is a more effective and cost-effective strategy: client reminder/recall, community-wide education, client or family incentives, reducing out-of-pocket expenses, or vaccination programs in schools?[23] This type of evidence points the researcher or practitioner toward the decision that *"specifically, this should be done"* (Type II Evidence).

Assessing the Quality and Limits of Evidence.   All scientific evidence is imperfect. As noted by Muir Gray, "The absence of excellent evidence does not make evidence-based decision making impossible; what is required is the best evidence available, not the best evidence possible."[24] As one attempts to determine the quality and usability of various types of evidence (particularly for Type II evidence), it useful to understand and apply established methods. For example, developers of the *Guide to Community Preventive Services* have adopted an approach for evaluating intervention effectiveness that takes into account both study design and study execution.[25] Several general criteria are useful in assessing the quality of a particular finding or piece of public health research (Table 1–4).[26, 27] These issues are discussed further in Chapters 2 and 3.

Table 1–4. Considerations for Evaluating the Quality of Public Health Research Findings

Less Certain Criteria	*More Certain Criteria*
One of a few observations	Many observations
Anecdote or case reports	Scientific study
Not published or peer-reviewed	Published in peer-reviewed journal
Not previously reported	Reproduces findings from other studies
Nonhuman subjects	Human subjects
Results not related to hypotheses	Results related to tested hypotheses
No limitations mentioned	Limitations mentioned
Not compared to previous results	Relationship to previous studies discussed

Sources: Nelson[26] and Riegelman[27]

Who Generates and Interprets Evidence?   Enhanced information technologies have made research findings, data, and other public health information more widely accessible to professional audiences, policy makers, and the general public. For example, the U.S. federal government and many state and local public health agencies now provide descriptive epidemiologic data on the World Wide Web. On balance, this proliferation of information is a highly positive development. To effectively utilize the vast array of data and program information, however, practitioners need an understanding of the types of data bases available, knowledge of their contents, and the ability to effectively access relevant information.[28] There are quick and effective ways of converting quantitative data into usable information for health policy makers, voluntary health advocates, and other decision makers.[29]

When Evidence Is Not Enough.   It is important to note that there is a cultural and geographical bias regarding the use and usefulness of evidence in the published literature.[30] Particularly in developing countries, much of the evidence base is unpublished. In fact, in many areas of the world, it may be a luxury to have the resources necessary for program evaluations that lead to externally valid scientific information. Even in more developed countries, including the United States, the data available through websites and official organizations many not adequately represent populations of interest. For example, the Behavioral Risk Factor Surveillance System is the world's largest telephone survey, yet it will not adequately represent subpopulations of communities with a higher likelihood of lacking telephones. Considerable effort is needed to better understand the criteria for evidence that should be applied in such settings.

Community-based participatory approaches also present challenges when utilizing evidence-based approaches. In these approaches, practitioners, academicians, and community members collaboratively define issues of concern, develop strategies for intervention, and evaluate the outcomes. It is, therefore, more difficult to begin a participatory program with preconceived notions of what the evidence dictates.

KEY CHARACTERISTICS OF EVIDENCE-BASED DECISION MAKING

It is useful to consider several overarching, common characteristics of an evidence-based approach to public health practice. These notions are expanded upon in other chapters.

Box 1–1. Tobacco Control in California

In the field of tobacco control, decades of research and thousands of epidemiologic studies comprise the evidence establishing cigarette smoking as the "single most important preventable cause of premature death."[31] Economic studies have shown that increased tobacco taxes are an important tool for decreasing tobacco consumption.[37] To address the issue, California voters passed an earmarked tobacco excise tax in 1988.[32] California raised the excise tax on cigarettes by 25 cents per pack and placed an initial tax of 42 cents on other tobacco products, with the rate on other tobacco products adjusted annually by the State Board of Equalization. This effort launched one of the most intensive and aggressive public health interventions ever undertaken.[34] This excise tax and media campaign was effective in sharply accelerating the drop in both sales of cigarettes and in smoking (for 1988–1993, double the rate expected based on the 1974–1987 trend). The program has also been associated with a reduction in deaths from heart disease in California.[35] However, in the period 1994–1996, the decline in smoking slowed, suggesting that sustained public health efforts are needed to maintain momentum for reduced smoking.[36]

Intervention Approaches Are Based on the Best Possible Science

As one evaluates Type II evidence, it is useful to understand where to turn for the best possible scientific evidence. A starting point is the scientific literature and guidelines developed by expert panels. In addition, preliminary findings from researchers and practitioners are often presented at regional, national, and international professional meetings. In Box 1–1, the decision to conduct a comprehensive tobacco control intervention was based on thousands of epidemiologic studies showing the causal associations between smoking and numerous health outcomes.[31] This large body of evidence has led to effective intervention strategies.[32–37]

Problem Solving Is Multidisciplinary

Effective problem solving in public health often requires expertise from individuals with diverse experiences and educational background. The full range of public health disciplines relies on professionals in management and administration, epidemiology, biostatistics, behavioral science, environmental health, and health economics.

Theory and Systematic Program Planning Approaches Are Used

When an approach is decided upon, a variety of planning frameworks and be-havioral science theories can be applied. As an example, ecological, or systems models are increasingly used in which "appropriate changes in the social envi-ronment will produce changes in individuals, and the support of individuals in a population is seen as essential for implementing environmental changes."[38] These models point to the importance of addressing problems at multiple levels and stress the interaction and integration of factors within and across all levels—in-dividual, interpersonal, community, organizational, and governmental. The goal is to create a healthy community environment that provides health-promoting in-formation and social support to enable people to live healthier lifestyles.[39] Effec-tive interventions are most often grounded in health-behavior theory.[40]

Sound Evaluation Principles Are Followed

Too often in public health, programs and policies are implemented without much attention to systematic evaluation. In addition, even when programs are ineffec-tive, they are sometimes continued because of historical or political considera-tions. Evaluation plans must be laid early in program development and should include both formative and outcome evaluation. As described in Box 1–2, an injury control program was appropriately discontinued after its effectiveness was evaluated. This program evaluation also illustrates the use of both qualitative and quantitative data in framing an evaluation.[41]

Results Are Disseminated to Others Who Need to Know

When a program or policy has been implemented, or when final results are known, others in public health can rely on findings to enhance their own use of evidence in decision making. Dissemination may occur to health professionals via the scientific literature, to the general public via the media, to policy makers through personal meetings and to public health professionals through training courses. Effective interventions are needed in a variety of settings, including schools, worksites, health care settings, and broader community environments.[42]

AN APPROACH TO INCREASING THE USE OF EVIDENCE IN PUBLIC HEALTH PRACTICE

In this section, a six-stage, sequential framework to promote greater use of evidence in day-to-day decision making is briefly described (Figure 1–2).[8] It is

---

Box 1–2. Example: Injury Prevention in Missouri

A Missouri program was designed to decrease motor vehicle injuries and deaths among children. In addressing this issue, the Missouri legislature enacted a child restraint law in 1984. The law required children younger than age 4 to travel in an approved safety seat in the front seat of a vehicle or in either a safety seat or seatbelt in the back seat. Even eight years after enactment, compliance was estimated at only 50%.[41] In response to concerns of health care providers and safety organizations, the Missouri Department of Health began the Take a Seat, Please! (TASP) Program in 1992, modeled after a similar program from Virginia. In TASP, volunteers were provided with business-reply postcards on which they could report the license plate number of a vehicle in which a child was not properly restrained. The owner of the vehicle was then sent a letter from the health department stating that the recipient had been observed, where and when the observation had taken place, information on child passenger safety, and program information through a toll-free number. Two years after implementation, the TASP program was evaluated through a telephone survey of participants and observational studies in child care centers.[41] The findings showed little evidence of program effectiveness; therefore, it was discontinued in September 1995. Similar approaches have been adopted in at least 15 other states with little supporting evidence of effectiveness.

---

important to note that this process is seldom a strictly prescriptive or linear one, but should include numerous feedback "loops" and processes that are common in many program planning models.[43] Each of these stages is discussed in more detail in subsequent chapters.

Develop an Initial Statement of the Issue

The practitioner should begin by developing a concise statement of the issue or problem being considered. To build support for any issue (with an organization, policy makers, or a funding agency), the issue must be clearly articulated. This problem definition stage has some similarities to the beginning steps in a strategic planning process, which often involves describing the mission, internal strengths and weaknesses, external opportunities and threats, and the vision for the future.[44, 45] It is often helpful to describe gaps between the current status of a program or organization and the desired goals. The key components of an issue statement include the health condition or risk factor being considered, the population(s) affected, the size and scope of the problem, prevention opportunities, and potential stakeholders.

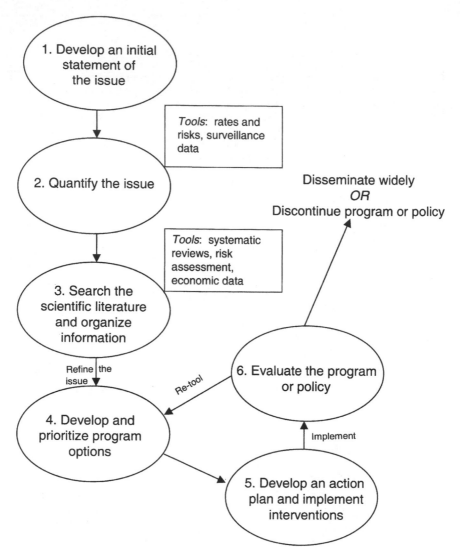

FIGURE 1–2. A sequential framework for enhancing evidence-based public health (adapted from Brownson et al.[8]).

Quantify the Issue

After developing a working description of the public health issue of interest, it is often useful to identify sources of existing data. Such descriptive data may be available from ongoing vital statistics data (birth/death records), surveillance systems, special surveys, or from national studies.

Descriptive studies can take several forms. In public health, the most common type of descriptive study involves a survey of a scientifically valid sample (a representative cross section) of the population of interest. These cross-sectional studies are not intended to change health status (as an intervention would), but rather they serve to quantify the prevalence of behaviors, characteristics, exposures, and diseases at some point (or period) of time in a defined population. This information can be valuable for understanding the scope of the public health problem at hand. Descriptive studies commonly provide information on patterns of occurrence according to such attributes as person (e.g., age, gender, ethnicity), place (e.g., county of residence), and time (e.g., seasonal variation in disease patterns). Additionally, under certain circumstances, cross-sectional data can provide information for use in the design of analytic studies (e.g., baseline data to evaluate the effectiveness of a public health intervention).

Search the Scientific Literature and Organize Information

Once the issue to be considered has been clearly defined, the practitioner needs to become knowledgeable about previous or ongoing efforts to address the issue. This should include a systematic approach to identify, retrieve, and evaluate relevant reports on scientific studies, panels, and conferences related to the defined topic of interest. The most common method for initiating this investigation is a formal literature review. There are many databases available to facilitate such a review. Most common among them for public health purposes are MED-LARS, MEDLINE, PubMed, PsycInfo, Current Contents, HealthSTAR, and CancerLit. These databases can be subscribed to by an organization, can selectively be found on the Internet, or sometimes can be accessed by the public through institutions (such as the National Library of Medicine (http://www.nlm.nih.gov), the Combined Health Information Database (http://chid.nih.gov), universities, and public libraries). There also are many organizations that maintain Internet sites that can be useful for identifying relevant information, including many state health departments, the Centers for Disease Control and Prevention, and the National Institutes of Health. It is important to remember that not all interventions (Type II) studies will be found in the published literature.

Develop and Prioritize Program Options

Based largely on the first three steps, a variety of health program or policy options are examined. The list of options can be developed from a variety of sources. The initial review of the scientific literature can sometimes highlight various intervention options. More often, expert panels provide program or policy recommendations on a variety of issues. Summaries of available evidence are often available in systematic reviews[46] and guidelines.[46–48] There are several assumptions or contexts underlying any development of options. These considerations focus in five main areas: political/regulatory, economic, social values, demographic, and technological.[45]

In particular, it is important to assess and monitor the political process when developing health policy options. To do so, "stakeholder" input may be useful. The stakeholder for a policy might be the health policy maker, whereas the stakeholder for a coalition-based community intervention might be a community member. In the case of health policies, supportive policy makers can frequently provide advice regarding timing of policy initiatives, methods for framing the issues, strategies for identifying sponsors, and ways to develop support among the general public. In the case of a community intervention, additional planning data may include key informant interviews, focus groups, or coalition member surveys.[49] Other tools of modern public health that are helpful in this and the following stage include social marketing and media advocacy.[50, 51]

Develop an Action Plan and Implement Interventions

This aspect of the process again deals largely with strategic planning issues. Once an option has been selected, a set of goals and objectives should be developed. A goal is a long-term desired change in the status of a priority health need, and an objective is a short-term, measurable, specific activity that leads toward achievement of a goal. The course of action describes how the goals and objectives will be achieved, what resources are required, and how responsibility for achieving objectives will be assigned.

Evaluate the Program or Policy

In simple terms, evaluation is the determination of the degree to which program or policy goals and objectives are met. If they follow any research design, most public health programs and policies are often evaluated through "quasi-experimental" designs, i.e., those lacking random assignment to intervention and comparison groups. In general, the strongest evaluation designs acknowledge the roles of both quantitative and qualitative evaluation. Furthermore, evaluation designs need to be flexible and sensitive enough to assess intermediate changes, even those that fall short of changes in behavior. Genuine change takes place incrementally over time, in ways that are often not visible to those too close to the intervention.

The six-stage framework of evidence-based public health summarized in this chapter is similar to an eight-step approach recently described by Jenicek.[7] An additional logical step focuses on teaching others how to practice evidence-based public health.[7] In Figure 1–2, this function is captured within the category of dissemination.

BARRIERS TO MORE EXTENSIVE USE OF EVIDENCE IN DECISION MAKING

There are several barriers to more effective use of data and analytic processes in decision making (Table 1–5). Possible approaches for overcoming these barriers have been discussed by others.[4, 52, 53] Leadership is needed from public health practitioners on the need and importance of evidence-based decision making. Such leadership is evident in training programs, such as the regional leadership network for public health practitioners[54] and the efforts underway to develop evidence-based guidelines for interventions.[47, 55, 56] To address the gap between curricula in academic institutions and "real world" needs, the Public Health Faculty/Agency Forum developed a useful set of universal and discipline-specific competencies and recommendations.[57]

Table 1–5. Potential Barriers and Solutions for Use of Evidence-Based Decision Making in Public Health

Barrier	Solution
Lack of leadership in setting a clear and focused agenda for evidence-based approaches	Commitment from all levels of public health leaders to increase the use of effective public health interventions
Lack of a view of the long-term "horizon" for program implementation and evaluation	Adoption and adherence to causal frameworks and formative evaluation plans
External (including political) pressures drive the process away from an evidence-based approach	Systematic communication and dissemination strategies
Inadequate training in key public health disciplines	Wider dissemination of new and established training programs, including use of distance learning technologies
Lack of time to gather information, analyze data, and review the literature for evidence	Enhanced skills for efficient analysis and review of the literature, computer searching abilities, ListServs
Lack of comprehensive, up-to-date information on the effectiveness of programs and policies	Increased dissemination of guidelines in clinical and population-based strategies
Lack of data on the effectiveness of certain public health interventions for special populations[a]	Increased funding for applied public health research; better dissemination of findings

[a]Special populations are defined as groups that have not been widely studied for a particular health condition or intervention, e.g., certain racial/ethnic populations or women.

SUMMARY

Current scientific and technologic advances provide unprecedented opportunities for public health professionals to improve their practice. To take full advantage of new tools, continued skill enhancement will be necessary. Training programs must account for the needs in public health practice, and practicing professionals should develop at least a basic understanding of analytic methods and ways of accurately assimilating a large body of scientific literature. Many of the issues introduced in this chapter can aid in this understanding and will subsequently be covered in more detail. It is noteworthy that, without significant attention to application and evidence-based approaches, research advances remain largely "on the shelf," and public health benefits are not conferred to communities in need.[58] A combination of scientific evidence, as well as values and resources, should enter into decision making (Figure 1–3). More effective public health practice will result from synthesis of scientific skills, enhanced communication, common sense, and political acumen.

This chapter has briefly summarized the rationale for evidence-based public health. Several important points were described:

- Lessons for public health can be learned from evidence-based approaches that have been adopted in medicine.
- Evidence is limited for many public health interventions, yet approaches should be based on the best possible science, be multidisciplinary, and center on sound planning and evaluation methods.

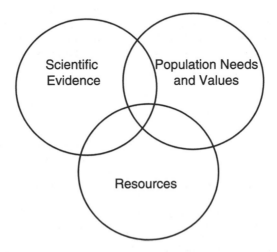

FIGURE 1–3. Broad considerations for enhancing decision making in public health (adapted and modified from Muir Gray[24]).

- A systematic approach to evidence-based decision making in public health is likely to improve practice.
- Barriers and limitations should be proactively addressed in a variety of public health settings.

SUGGESTED READINGS AND WEBSITES

Readings

Brownson RC, Gurney JG, Land G. Evidence-based decision making in public health. *Journal of Public Health Management and Practice* 1999;5:86–97.

Guyatt G, Rennie D, eds. *Users' Guides to the Medical Literature. A Manual for Evidence-Based Clinical Practice.* Chicago: American Medical Association Press, 2002.

Jenicek M. Epidemiology, evidence-based medicine, and evidence-based public health. *Journal of Epidemiology* 1997;7:187–197.

Muir Gray JA. *Evidence-Based Healthcare: How to Make Health Policy and Management Decisions.* New York and Edinburgh: Churchill Livingstone, 1997.

Sackett DL, Rosenberg WMC, Gray JAM, Haynes RB, Richardson WS. Evidence based medicine: what it is and what it isn't. *British Medical Journal* 1996;312:71–72.

Selected Websites

American Public Health Association <http://www.apha.org/>. The American Public Health Association (APHA) is the oldest and largest organization of public health professionals in the world, representing more than 50,000 members from over 50 occupations of public health. The Association and its members have been influencing policies and setting priorities in public health since 1872. The APHA site also provides links to many other useful websites.

Guide to Community Preventive Services <http://www.thecommunityguide.org>. Under the auspices of the U.S. Public Health Service, a Task Force on Community Preventive Services (the Task Force) is developing a *Guide to Community Preventive Services* (the *Guide*). The *Guide* will summarize what is known about the effectiveness of population-based interventions for prevention and control.

Guide to Clinical Preventive Services, Second Edition <http://odphp.osophs.dhhs.gov/pubs/guidecps>. This report is intended for primary care clinicians: physicians, nurses, nurse practitioners, physician assistants, other allied health professionals, and students. It provides recommendations for clinical practice on preventive interventions-screening tests, counseling interventions, immunizations, and chemoprophylactic regimens-for the prevention of more than 80 target conditions. The recommendations in each chapter reflect a standardized review of current scientific evidence and include a summary of published clinical research regarding the clinical effectiveness of each preventive service.

Partnership for Prevention <http://www.prevent.org/>. Working to emphasize disease prevention and health promotion in national policy and practice, Partnership for Prevention is a membership association of corporations, nonprofits, and state health departments. It provides high-quality information about prevention to policy makers such as members of Congress, corporate leaders, and state and local health officials.

Public Health, Department of Health Services, Victoria, Australia <http://www.dhs. vic.gov.au/phd/>. The Public Health Division is committed to improving the health and well being of the whole population of Victoria in a way that addresses social inequality and the underlying determinants of health, empowers families and communities, uses evidence-based research, and ensures value for money.

The United Kingdom Public Health Association <http://www.ukpha.org.uk/>. The United Kingdom Public Health Association is an independent UK-wide voluntary association, bringing together individuals and organizations from all sectors, who share a commitment to promoting the public's health. It is a membership-based organization that aims to promote the development of healthy public policy at all levels of government and across all sectors and to support those working in public health either professionally or in a voluntary capacity.

US Census <http://www.census.gov/>. A large collection of timely, relevant, and quality data about the people and economy of the United States.

REFERENCES

1. National Center for Health Statistics. *Health, United States, 2000 With Adolescent Health Chartbook.* Hyattsville, MD: Centers for Disease Control and Prevention, National Center for Health Statistics, 2000.
2. Centers for Disease Control and Prevention. *Public Health in the New American Health System. Discussion Paper.* Atlanta, GA: Centers for Disease Control and Prevention, March, 1993.
3. U.S. Dept. of Health and Human Services. *Healthy People 2010. Volume II. Conference Edition.* Washington, DC: US Department of Health and Human Services, 2000.
4. IOM. Committee for the Study of the Future of Public Health. *The Future of Public Health.* Washington, DC: National Academy Press; 1988.
5. Bialek R. Building the science base for public health practice. *Journal of Public Health Management and Practice* 2000;6(5):51–58.
6. Jewell EJ, Abate F, eds. *The New Oxford American Dictionary.* New York: Oxford University Press, 2001.
7. Jenicek M. Epidemiology, evidence-based medicine, and evidence-based public health. *Journal of Epidemiology* 1997;7:187–197.
8. Brownson RC, Gurney JG, Land G. Evidence-based decision making in public health. *Journal of Public Health Management and Practice* 1999;5:86–97.
9. Schmid TL, Pratt M, Howze E. Policy as intervention: Environmental and policy approaches to the prevention of cardiovascular disease. *American Journal of Public Health* 1995;85(9):1207–1211.
10. Cheadle A, Wagner E, Koepsell T, Kristal A, Patrick D. Environmental indicators: A tool of evaluating community-based health-promotion programs. *American Journal of Preventive Medicine* 1992;8:345–350.
11. Evidence-Based Medicine Working Group. Evidence-based medicine. A new approach to teaching the practice of medicine. *Journal of the American Medical Association* 1992;17:2420–2425.

12. Guyatt G, Rennie D, eds. *Users' Guides to the Medical Literature. A Manual for Evidence-Based Clinical Practice*. Chicago, IL: American Medical Association Press, 2002.
13. Sackett DL, Rosenberg WMC, Gray JAM, Haynes RB, Richardson WS. Evidence based medicine: What it is and what it isn't. *British Medical Journal* 1996;312:71–72.
14. Taubes G. Looking for the evidence in medicine. *Science* 1996;272:22–24.
15. Sackett DL, Rosenberg WMC. The need for evidence-based medicine. *Journal of the Royal Society of Medicine* 1995;88:620–624.
16. Rosenberg W, Donald A. Evidence-based medicine: An approach to clinical problem solving. *British Medical Journal* 1995;310:1122–1126.
17. Ellrodt G, Cook DJ, Lee J, Cho M, Hung D, Weingarten S. Evidence-based disease management. *Journal of the American Medical Association* 1997;278:1687–1692.
18. Field MJ, Lohr KN, eds. *Clinical Practice Guidelines: Directions for a New Program*. Washington, DC: National Academy Press, 1990.
19. Woolf SH, DiGuiseppi CG, Atkins D, Kamerow DB. Developing evidence-based clinical practice guidelines: Lessons learned by the U.S. Preventive Services Task Force. *Annual Review of Public Health* 1996;17:511–538.
20. Shekelle PG, Woolf SF, Eccles M, Grimshaw J. Clinical guidelines: Developing guidelines. *British Medical Journal* 1999;318:593–596.
21. Turnock BJ. *Public Health: What It Is and How It Works*. 2nd ed. Gaithersburg, MD: Aspen Publishers, Inc., 2001.
22. Thacker SB, Koplan JP, Taylor WR, Hinman AR, Katz MF, Roper WL. Assessing prevention effectiveness using data to drive program decisions. *Public Health Reports* 1994;109:187–194.
23. Task Force on Community Preventive Services. Recommendations regarding interventions to improve vaccination coverage in children, adolescents, and adults. *American Journal of Preventive Medicine* 2000;18(1S):92–96.
24. Muir Gray JA. *Evidence-Based Healthcare: How to Make Health Policy and Management Decisions*. New York and Edinburgh: Churchill Livingstone, 1997.
25. Briss PA, Zaza S, Pappaioanou M, et al. Developing an evidence-based Guide to Community Preventive Services—methods. The Task Force on Community Preventive Services. *American Journal of Preventive Medicine* 2000;18(1 Suppl):35–43.
26. Nelson DE. Tranlating public health data. In: Nelson DE, Brownson RC, Remington PL, Parvanta C, eds. *Communicating Public Health Information Effectively: A Guide for Public Health Practitioners*. Washington, DC: American Public Health Association, (in press).
27. Riegelman RK. *Studying a Study and Testing a Test*. 4th ed. Philadelphia: Lippincott Williams & Wilkins, 2000.
28. Glasziou P, Longbottom H. Evidence-based public health practice. *Australian and New Zealand Journal of Public Health* 1999;23(4):436–440.
29. Nelson DE. Assessing the science, locating information, and translating data. In: Nelson DE, Brownson RC, Remington PL, Parvanta C, eds. *Communicating Public Health Information Effectively: A Guide for Public Health Practitioners*. Washington, DC: American Public Health Association, (in press).
30. McQueen D. Strengthing the evidence base for health promotion. Paper presented at the Fifth Global Conference for Health Promotion. Health Promotion: Bridging the Equity Gap, Mexico City, Mexico, June 5–9, 2000.
31. U.S. Dept. of Health and Human Services. *Reducing the Health Consequences of*

Smoking—25 Years of Progress: A Report of the Surgeon General. Vol DHHS publication (CDC) 89–8411. Rockville, MD: U.S. Dept. of Health and Human Services, Public Health Service, Centers for Disease Control, Center for Chronic Disease Prevention and Health Promotion, Office on Smoking and Health; 1989.

32. Bal D, Kizer K, Felten P, Mozar H, Niemeyer D. Reducing tobacco consumption in California: Development of a statewide anti-tobacco use campaign. *JAMA.* 1990;264: 1570–1574.

33. Centers for Disease Control and Prevention. *Best Practices for Comprehensive Tobacco Control Programs.* Atlanta, GA: Centers for Disease Control and Prevention, National Center for Chronic Disease Prevention and Health Promotion, Office on Smoking and Health; August 1999.

34. Elder JP, Edwards CC, Conway TL, et al. Independent evaluation of the California tobacco education program. *Public Health Reports* 1996;111:353–358.

35. Fichtenberg CM, Glantz SA. Association of the California Tobacco Control Program with declines in cigarette consumption and mortality from heart disease. *New England Journal of Medicine* 2000;343(24):1772–1777.

36. Pierce JP, Gilpin EA, Emery SL, et al. Has the California tobacco control program reduced smoking? *Journal of the American Medical Association* 1998;280(10):893–899.

37. Sweanor D, Ballin S, Corcoran RD, et al. Report of the Tobacco Policy Research Study Group on tobacco pricing and taxation in the United States. *Tobacco Control 1992.* Vol 1(suppl); 1992:S31–S36.

38. McLeroy KR, Bibeau D, Steckler A, Glanz K. An ecological perspective on health promotion programs. *Health Education Quarterly* 1988;15:351–377.

39. Stokols D. Translating social ecological theory into guidelines for community health promotion. *American Journal of Health Promotion* 1996;10(4):282–298.

40. Rimer BK, Glanz DK, Rasband G. Searching for evidence about health education and health behavior interventions. *Health Education and Health Behavior* 2001; 28(2):231–248.

41. Land G, Romeis JC, Gillespie KN, Denny S. Missouri's Take a Seat, Please! and Program Evaluation. *Journal of Public Health Management and Practice* 1997;3(6): 51–58.

42. Sallis JF, Owen N, Fotheringham MJ. Behavioral epidemiology: A systematic framework to classify phases of research on health promotion and disease prevention. *Annals of Behavioral Medicine* 2000;22(4):294–298.

43. U.S. Dept. of Health and Human Services. *Planned Approach to Community Health: Guide for the Local Coordinator.* Atlanta: Centers for Disease Control and Prevention, 1998.

44. Bryson JM. *Strategic Planning for Public and Nonprofit Organizations. A Guide to Strengthening and Sustaining Organizational Achievement.* San Francisco: Jossey-Bass Publishers, 1995.

45. Ginter PM, Duncan WJ, Capper SA. Keeping strategic thinking in strategic planning: macro-environmental analysis in a state health department of public health *Public Health* 1992;106:253–269.

46. Mulrow C, Cook D, eds. *Systematic Reviews. Synthesis of Best Evidence for Health Care Decisions.* Philadelphia: American College of Physicians; 1998.

47. Truman BI, Smith-Akin CK, Hinman AR, et al. Developing the guide to community preventive services—overview and rationale. *American Journal of Preventive Medicine* 2000;18(1S):18–26.

48. U.S. Preventive Services Task Force. *Guide to Clinical Preventive Services*. 2nd ed. Baltimore: Williams & Wilkins, 1996.
49. Florin P, Stevenson J. Identifying training and technical assistance needs in community coalitions: A developmental approach. *Health Education Research* 1993;8: 417–432.
50. Doner L, Siegel M. Public health marketing. In: Novick LF and Mays GP, eds. *Public Health Administration. Principles for Population-Based Management*. Gaithersburg, MD: Aspen Publishers, Inc., 2001, pp. 474–509.
51. Wallack L, Dorfman L, Jernigan D, Themba M. *Media Advocacy and Public Health: Power for Prevention*. Newbury Park, CA: Sage, 1993.
52. Brownson RC, Kreuter MW. Future trends affecting public health: Challenges and opportunities. *Journal of Public Health Management and Practice* 1997;3:49–60.
53. IOM. Committee on Public Health. *Healthy Communities: New Partnerships for the Future of Public Health*. Washington, DC: National Academy Press; 1996.
54. Gordon RL, Baker EL, Roper WL, Omenn GS. Prevention and the reforming U.S. health care system: changing roles and responsibilities for public health. *Annual Review of Public Health* 1996;17:489–509.
55. Breslow L. The future of public health: Prospects in the United States for the 1990s. *Annual Review of Public Health* 1990;11:1–28.
56. Zaza S, Lawrence RS, Mahan CS, et al. Scope and organization of the Guide to Community Preventive Services. *American Journal of Preventive Medicine* 2000; 18(1S):27–34.
57. Sorensen AA, Bialek RG, eds. *The Public Health Faculty/Agency Forum: Linking Graduate Education and Practice: Final Report*. Gainesville, FL: University Press of Florida, 1991.
58. Institute of Medicine. *Linking research to public health practice. A review of the CDC's program of Centers for Research and Demonstration of Health Promotion and Disease Prevention*. Washington, D.C.: National Academy Press, 1997.

2

Assessing Scientific Evidence for Public Health Action

> It is often necessary to make a decision on the basis of information sufficient for action but insufficient to satisfy the intellect.
> —Immanuel Kant

In most areas of public health and clinical practice, decisions on when to intervene and which program or policy to implement are not simple and straightforward. These decisions are often based on three fundamental questions: (1) Should public health action be taken to address a particular public health issue (primarily based on Type I evidence)? (2) What action should be taken (primarily based on Type II evidence)? and (3) How can a particular program or policy most effectively be implemented and evaluated? This chapter primarily explores the first question. That is, it focuses on several key considerations in evaluating scientific evidence and determining when a scientific basis exists for some type of public health action. It deals largely with the interpretation of epidemiologic studies that seek to identify health risks associated with preventable morbidity and mortality. The second and third questions are explored in more detail in later chapters.

BACKGROUND

In this era when public and media interest in health issues is intense, the reasons for not taking action based on an individual research study, especially if it was carefully designed, successfully conducted, and properly analyzed and interpreted, need to be emphasized. Public health research is incremental, with a body of scientific evidence building up over years or decades. Therefore, while individual studies may contribute substantially to public health decision making, a single study rarely constitutes a strong basis for action. The example in Box

---

Box 2–1. Toxic Shock Syndrome in the United States

In the case of an infectious agent transmitted by a fomite (i.e., an inanimate object that may harbor a pathogen), the illness known as toxic shock syndrome was reported to the Centers for Disease Control by individual physicians and five state health departments beginning in October 1979.[35] Toxic shock syndrome began with high fever, vomiting, and profuse watery diarrhea and progressed to hypotensive shock. Among the first 55 cases, the case fatality ratio was 13%. The bacterium *Staphylococcus aureus* was found to be responsible for the syndrome. Through a nationwide case-control study of 52 cases and 52 matched controls, the mode of transmission was determined to be the use of high absorbency (fluid capacity) tampons in women.[36] The findings of epidemiologic studies led to public health recommendations to women regarding safe use of tampons, a voluntary removal of the Rely brand, and subsequent lowering of absorbency of all brands of tampons.[37] These actions in turn led to substantial reductions in the incidence of toxic shock syndrome since the early observations of the association between tampon use and toxic shock syndrome.

2–1 regarding toxic shock syndrome is unusual since rapid action was taken based on a small but convincing body of scientific evidence.

When considering the science, strong evidence from epidemiologic (and other) studies may suggest that control measures should be taken. Conversely, evidence may be equivocal, so that taking action would be premature. Often the strength of evidence is suggestive, but not conclusive; yet one has to make a decision about the desirability of taking action. Here, other questions come to mind:

- How serious are the consequences of taking some action or no action, and what other impact will the course of action have?
- Will the action reduce the frequency and/or severity of a serious disease?
- Are there few (if any) adverse effects of intervention?
- Is the action inexpensive and/or cost-effective?

If the answer to the final three questions is "yes," then the decision to take action is straightforward. In practice, unfortunately, decisions are seldom so simple.

EXAMINING A BODY OF SCIENTIFIC EVIDENCE

As practitioners, researchers, and policy makers committed to improving population health, we have a natural tendency to scrutinize the scientific literature for new findings that would serve as the basis for prevention or intervention programs.[1] In fact, the main motivation for conducting research should be to stimulate appropriate public health action. Adding to this inclination to intervene may be claims from investigators regarding the critical importance of their findings, media interpretation of the findings as the basis for immediate action, and community support for responding to the striking new research findings with new or modified programs. The importance of community action in motivating public health efforts was shown recently in the Long Island Breast Cancer Study. Community advocates in Long Island raised concerns about the high incidence of breast cancer and possible linkages with environmental chemicals and radiation. A series of studies are being conducted by the New York State Health Department, along with scientists from universities and the National Institutes of Health. In each Long Island-area county, breast cancer incidence increased over a ten-year period, while mortality from breast cancer decreased.[2] To date, a case-control study has shown that women living closer to chemical facilities have a higher risk of postmenopausal breast cancer, but linkages with specific environmental agents have not been demonstrated and several detailed studies are ongoing.

Finding Scientific Evidence

Chapter 6 describes systematic methods for seeking out credible, peer-reviewed scientific evidence. Modern information technologies have made searching the scientific literature quick and accessible. There are also hundreds of websites that summarize research and provide ready access to surveillance data. The ready access to information may also present a paradox, in that access to more information is assumed to be productive, yet bad science and bad advice are also found in the myriad of information on various topics. Often, various tools are helpful in examining an entire body of evidence, rather than reviewing the literature study-by-study. These summary approaches, described in Chapter 3, include systematic reviews of the literature, evidence-based guidelines, summaries of best practices, and economic evaluations.

The Roles of Peer Review and Publication Bias

In assessing evidence, it is important to understand the role of peer review. Peer review is the process of reviewing research proposals, manuscripts submitted for publication by journals, and abstracts submitted for presentation at scientific meetings. These materials are judged for scientific and technical merit by other scientists in the same field.[3] Reviewers are commonly asked to comment on such issues as the scientific soundness of the methods used, originality, relevance, and appropriateness of a scientific article to the audience. Although peer review has numerous limitations, including a large time commitment, complexity, and expense, it remains the closest approximation to a gold standard when determining the merits of scientific endeavor.

Publication bias is the higher likelihood for journal editors to publish positive or "new" findings in contrast to negative studies or those that do not yield statistically significant results. Studies have shown that positive findings tend to get published more often and more quickly.[4] There are numerous possible reasons for publication bias, including researchers' tendency to submit positive rather than negative studies, peer reviewers who are more likely to recommend publication of positive studies, and journal editors who favor publication of positive studies.[5] The net effect of publication bias may be an overrepresentation of false positive findings in the literature. It is also important to be aware of potential publication bias when reading or conducting meta-analyses that rely solely on the published literature and do not seek out unpublished studies. When a sufficient number of studies is available, funnel plots may be an effective method by which to determine whether publication bias is present in a particular body of evidence.[5, 6] Figure 2–1 presents hypothetical data showing the effects of publication bias. In the plot on the right-hand side, smaller studies are represented in the literature only when they tend to show a positive effect. Thus, the left side of the inverted funnel is missing, and publication bias may be present.

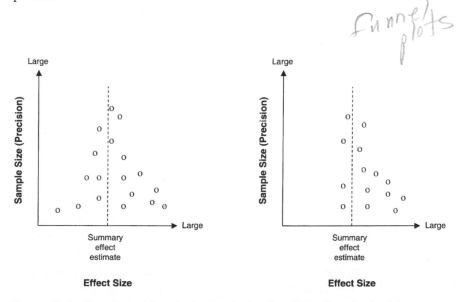

FIGURE 2–1. Hypothetical funnel plots illustrating the effect of publication bias.

STUDY DESIGN ISSUES: QUALITY AND GENERALIZABILITY

Public health information for decision making is founded upon science, and science is based on the collection, analysis, and interpretation of data.[7] Data in public health are generally derived from two overlapping sources: research studies and public health surveillance systems. Here, we focus on information from research studies; an emphasis on public health surveillance is provided in Chapter 3. Research studies are primarily conducted in four broad areas: (1) to understand the etiologies of health conditions (Does fruit and vegetable intake influence the risk of coronary heart disease?); (2) to determine whether public health interventions are successful in meeting their stated objectives for risk reduction (Is a media campaign to increase fruit and vegetable intake effective?); (3) to explore the links between interventions and etiology (Does an intervention that increases consumption of fruits and vegetable result in a decline in coronary heart disease incidence?); and (4) to develop and test new research methods (What are the most valid and reliable methods by which to measure fruit and vegetable consumption?).

The quality of the evidence from a given study can be assessed based on the study design, execution of the study (internal validity), and generalizability (external validity). In public health research, a variety of study designs is used to assess health risks and to measure intervention effectiveness. Commonly, these are not "true" experiments in which study participants are randomized to an intervention or control condition. These generally quasi-experimental or observational designs are described in Chapter 5. A hierarchy of designs shows that a randomized trial tends to be the strongest type of study, yet such a study is often not feasible in community settings (Table 2–1).[8] Interestingly, when summary results from the same topic were based on observational studies and on randomized controlled trials, the findings across study designs were remarkably similar.[9]

The quality of a study's execution can be determined by many different standards. Individual studies are often judged on the basis of their internal validity. While it is beyond the scope of this chapter to discuss these issues in detail, an overview of key issues is provided, along with entry points into a larger body of literature. For a study or program evaluation to be internally valid, the study and comparison groups should be selected and compared in a way that the observed differences in dependent variables are attributed to the hypothesized effects under study (apart from sampling error).[3] In other words, can the observed results be attributed to the risk factor being studied or intervention being implemented? These concepts are illustrated in Figure 2–2. In general, internal validity is threatened by all types of systematic error, and error rates are influenced by both study design and study execution. Systematic error occurs when

Table 2–1. Hierarchy of Study Designs

Suitability	Examples	Attributes
Greatest	Randomized group or individual trial; prospective cohort study; time series study with comparison group	Concurrent comparison groups and prospective measurement of exposure and outcome
Moderate	Case-control study; time series study without comparison group	All retrospective designs or multiple pre- or postmeasurements but no concurrent comparison group
Least	Cross-sectional study; case series; ecological study	Before-after studies with no comparison group or exposure and outcome measured in a single group at the same point in time

Source: Adapted from Briss et al., 2000.[8]

there is a tendency within a particular study to produce results that vary in a systematic way from the true values.[10] Dozens of specific types of bias have been identified. Among the most important are

1. Selection bias: error due to systematic differences in characteristics between those who take part in the study and those who do not[3]
2. Information bias: a flaw in measuring exposure or outcomes that results in different quality (accuracy) of information between study groups[3]
3. Confounding bias: distortion of the estimated effect of an exposure on an outcome, caused by the presence of an extraneous factor associated with both the exposure and the outcome[3]

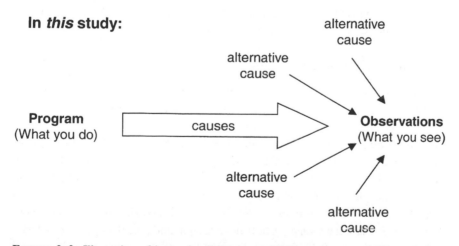

FIGURE 2–2. Illustration of internal validity in establishing a cause and effect relationship (*Source:* <http://trochim.human.cornell.edu/kb/>).

In ongoing work of the U.S. Public Health Service,[11, 12] study execution is assessed according to six categories, each of which may threaten internal validity: (1) study population and intervention descriptions; (2) sampling; (3) exposure and outcome measurement; (4) data analysis; (5) interpretation of results (including follow-up, bias, and confounding); and (6) other related factors.[8]

External validity, synonymous with generalizability, relates to whether a study can produce unbiased inferences to other populations beyond the subjects in the study.[3] Internal validity of a study is necessary for, but does not guarantee, external validity.[10] For example, are the findings from a study of middle-aged white males applicable to ethnically diverse women? In practice, multicenter studies among diverse populations, using similar methods, are sometimes conducted to enhance the likelihood of attaining external validity.

ASSESSING CAUSALITY IN PUBLIC HEALTH RESEARCH

Any intervention program or public health action is based on the presumption that the associations found in epidemiologic studies are causal rather than arising through bias or for some other spurious reason.[1] A cause of a disease is an event, condition, characteristic, or combination of factors that plays an important role in the development of the disease or health condition.[10] Unfortunately, in most instances in observational research, there is no opportunity to prove absolutely that an association is causal. Nonetheless, numerous frameworks have been developed that are useful in determining whether a cause-and-effect relationship exists between a particular risk factor and a given health outcome. This is one of the reasons for assembling experts to reach scientific consensus on various issues (discussed in Chapter 3).

Criteria for Assessing Causality

The earliest guidelines for assessing causality for infectious diseases were developed in the 1800s by Jacob Henle and Robert Koch. The Henle-Koch Postulates state that: (1) the agent must be shown to be present in every case of the disease by isolation in pure culture; (2) the agent must not be found in cases of other disease; (3) once isolated, the agent must be capable of reproducing the disease in experimental animals; and (4) the agent must be recovered from the experimental disease produced.[3, 13] These postulates have proven less useful in evaluating causality for more contemporary health conditions since most noninfectious diseases have long periods of induction and multifactorial causation.[14]

Subsequently, the U.S. Surgeon General,[15] Hill,[16] Susser,[17] and Rothman[18] have all provided insights into causal criteria, particularly in regard to causation of chronic diseases such as heart disease, cancer, and arthritis. Although criteria have sometimes been cited as checklists for assessing causality, they were intended as factors to consider when examining an association: they have value, but only as general guidelines. Several criteria relate to particular cases of refuting biases or drawing on nonepidemiologic evidence. These criteria have been discussed in detail elsewhere.[15-17, 19] In the end, belief in causality is based on an individual's judgment, and different individuals may in good faith reach different conclusions from the same available information. The six key issues below have been adapted from Hill[16] and Weed.[20] Each is described by a definition and a rule of evidence. These are also illustrated in Table 2–2 by examining two risk-factor/disease relationships.

1. *Consistency*

   Definition: The association is observed in studies in different settings and populations, using various methods.

   Rule of evidence: The likelihood of a causal association increases as the proportion of studies with similar (positive) results increases.

2. *Strength*

   Definition: This is defined by the size of the relative risk estimate. In some situations, meta-analytic techniques are used to provide an overall, summary risk estimate.

   Rule of evidence: The likelihood of a causal association increases as the summary relative risk estimate increases. Larger effect estimates are generally less likely to be explained by unmeasured bias or confounding.

3. *Temporality*

   Definition: This is perhaps the most important criterion for causality— some consider it an absolute condition. Temporality refers to the temporal relationship between the occurrence of the risk factor and the occurrence of the disease or health condition.

   Rule of evidence: The exposure (risk factor) must precede the disease.

4. *Dose–response relationship*

   Definition: The observed relationship between the dose of the exposure and the magnitude of the relative risk estimate.

   Rule of evidence: An increasing level of exposure (in intensity and/or time) increases the risk when hypothesized to do so.

5. *Biological plausibility*

   Definition: The available knowledge on the biological mechanism of action for the studied risk factor and disease outcome.

   Rule of evidence: There is not a standard rule of thumb except that the more likely the agent is biologically capable of influencing the disease, then the more probable that a causal relationship exists.

6. *Experimental evidence*
   Definition: The presence of findings from a prevention trial in which the factor of interest is removed from randomly assigned individuals.
   Rule of evidence: A positive result (i.e., reduction in a health condition) after removal of the risk factor is strong evidence that the factor is causal.

In practice, evidence for causality is often established through the elimination of noncausal explanations for an observed association. For example, consider the evidence that alcohol use may increase the risk of breast cancer.[1] A series of further studies might confirm that this relationship is internally valid and not a result of confounding or other biases. By whittling away alternative explanations, the hypothesis that asserts alcohol use causes breast cancer becomes increasingly credible. It is the job of researchers to propose and test noncausal explanations, so that when the association has withstood a series of such challenges, the case for causality is strengthened.

Since most associations involve unknown confounders, a key issue becomes the extent to which causal conclusions or public health recommendations should be delayed until all or nearly all potential confounders are discovered and/or better measured.[21] As noted earlier, those who argue that causality must be established with absolute certainty before interventions are attempted may fail to appreciate that their two alternatives—action and inaction—each have risks and benefits. When searching for causal relationships, researchers generally seek those that are modifiable and potentially amenable to some type of public health intervention. If researchers discovered that time of initiation of teen smoking was strongly related to the ethnicity of the teen and exposure to advertising, for example, the latter variable would be a likely target of intervention efforts.

RELATED ISSUES WHEN CONSIDERING PUBLIC HEALTH ACTION

In addition to understanding scientific causality and methods for accessing the published literature, several related issues are important to consider when weighing public health action.

Factors Influencing Decision Making in Public Health

There are many factors that influence decision making in public health (Table 2-3).[22] Some of these factors are under the control of the public health practitioner, whereas others are nearly impossible to modify. A group of experts may

Table 2–2. Degree to Which Causal Criteria Are Met for Two Contemporary Public Health Issues

Issue	Physical Activity and Coronary Heart Disease (CHD)	Extremely Low Frequency Electromagnetic Fields (EMFs) and Childhood Cancer[a]
Consistency	Approximately 50 studies since 1953; vast majority of studies show positive association	Based on a relatively small number of studies, the preponderance of the evidence favors a judgment of no association
Strength	Median relative risk of 1.9 for a sedentary lifestyle across studies, after controlling for other risk factors	Early studies showed relative risks in the range of 1.5 to 2.5. Most subsequent studies with larger sample sizes and more comprehensive exposure methods have not shown positive associations
Temporality	Satisfied, based on prospective cohort study design	Not satisfied; very difficult to assess because of ubiquitous exposure and the rarity of the disease
Dose–response relationship	Most studies show an inverse relationship between physical activity and risk of CHD	Since there is little biological guidance into what component(s) of EMF exposure may be problematic, exposure assessment is subject to a high degree of misclassification. True dose gradients are therefore very hard to classify reliably
Biological plausibility	Biological mechanisms are demonstrated, including: atherosclerosis, plasma/lipid changes, blood pressure, ischemia, and thrombosis	No direct cancer mechanism is yet known, as EMFs produce energy levels far too low to cause DNA damage or chemical reactions
Experimental evidence	Trials have not been conducted related to CHD but have been carried out for CHD intermediate factors such as blood pressure, lipoprotein profile, insulin sensitivity, and body fat	Numerous experimental studies of EMF exposure have been conducted to assess indirect mechanisms for carcinogenesis in animals and via in vitro cell models. The few positive findings to date have not been successfully reproduced in other laboratories

[a]Predominantly childhood leukemia and brain cancer.

Table 2–3. Factors Influencing Decision Making among Public Health Administrators, Policy Makers, and the General Public

Category	Influential Factor
Information	• Sound scientific basis, including knowledge of causality • Source (e.g., professional organization, government, mass media, friends)
Clarity of contents	• Formatting and framing • Perceived validity • Perceived relevance • Strength of the message (i.e., vividness)
Perceived values, preferences, beliefs	• Role of the decision maker • Economic background • Previous education • Personal experience or involvement • Political affiliation or political climate • Willingness to adopt innovations • Willingness to accept uncertainty • Willingness to accept risk • Ethical aspect of the decision
Context	• Culture • Lobbying • Timing • Media attention • Administrative, financial, or political constraints

Source: adapted from Bero et al., 1998.[22]

systematically assemble and present a persuasive body of scientific evidence such as recommendations for clinical or community-based interventions,[11, 12, 16, 23] but even when they convene in a rational and evidence-based manner, the process is imperfect, participants may disagree, and events may become politically charged, as noted in Table 2–3 and Box 2–2.[24] In addition, one may have little control over the timing of some major public health event (e.g., prostate cancer diagnosis in an elected leader) that may have a large impact on the awareness and behaviors of the general public and policy makers.

Assessing Population Burden

As noted earlier, many factors enter into decisions about public health interventions, including certainty of causality, validity, relevance, economics, and political climate (Table 2–3). Measures of burden may also contribute substantially to science-based decision making. The burden of infectious diseases, such as measles, has been primarily assessed through incidence, measured in case numbers or rates. For chronic or noninfectious diseases like cancer, burden can be measured in terms of morbidity, mortality, and disability. The choice of measure should depend on the characteristics of the condition being examined. For ex-

Box 2–2. Establishing Breast Cancer Screening Guidelines

Breast cancer screening guidance for women ages 40 to 49 years has been the subject of considerable debate and controversy. Breast cancer is the most common cancer type among U.S. women, accounting for 182,800 new cases and 40,800 annual deaths.[38] It is suggested that appropriate use of screening mammography may lower death rates due to breast cancer up to 30%. Official expert guidance from the U.S. government was first issued in 1977 when the National Cancer Institute (NCI) recommended annual mammography screening for women ages 50 and older but discouraged screening for younger women.[39] In 1980, the American Cancer Society dissented from this guidance and recommended a baseline mammogram for women at age 35 years and annual or biannual mammograms for women in their 40s.[40] The NCI and other professional organizations differed on recommendations for women in their 40s throughout the late 1980s and 1990s. To resolve disagreement, the director of the National Institutes of Health called for a Consensus Development Conference in January 1997. Based on evidence from randomized, controlled trials, the consensus group concluded that the available data did not support a blanket mammography recommendation for women in their 40s. The panel issued a draft statement that largely left the decision regarding screening up to the woman (Table 2–4).[41] This guidance led to widespread media attention and controversy. Within one week, the U.S. Senate passed a 98 to 0 vote resolution calling on the NCI to express unequivocal support for screening women in their 40s, and within 60 days, the NCI had issued a new recommendation.

ample, mortality rates are useful in reporting data on a fatal condition such as lung cancer. For a common, yet generally nonfatal condition such as arthritis, a measure of disability would be more useful (e.g., limitations in "activities of daily living"). When available, measures of the population burden of health conditions are extremely useful, e.g., quality-adjusted life years (QALYs) (see Chapter 3).

When assessing the scientific basis for a public health program or policy, quantitative considerations of preventable disease can help us make a rational choice. This can be thought of as "preventable burden." When presented with an array of potential causal factors for disease, we need to evaluate how much might be gained by reducing or eliminating each of the hazards. For example, can we predict in numerical terms the benefits that one or more interventions might yield in the community?

Epidemiologic measures, such as relative risk estimates indicate how strongly exposure and disease are associated, but they do not indicate directly the benefits that could be gained through modifying the exposure. Of still greater potential value is the incorporation of information on how common the exposure is. Although some exposures exert a powerful influence on individuals (i.e., a large relative risk), they are so rare that their public health impact is minimal. Conversely, some exposures have a modest impact but are so widespread that their elimination could have great benefit. To answer the question, "What proportion

Table 2–4. Chronology and Selected Statements from the Development of Consensus Breast Cancer Screening Guidelines for Women Aged 40 to 49 Years, 1997

Date	Source	Statement or Quote
January 23, 1997	NIH Consensus Development Panel (called for and co-sponsored by the National Cancer Institute)	Every woman should decide for herself "based not only on objective analysis of scientific evidence and consideration of her individual medical history, bus also on how she perceives and weighs each potential risk and benefits, the values she places on each and how she deals with uncertainty."
January 24, 1997	American Cancer Society	"The confusion surrounding the important question of whether women in their 40s should have regular mammograms had not been cleared up and perhaps was made even murkier by the recent announcement."
February 4, 1997	U.S. Senator Mikulski	"I could not believe when an NIH advisory panel decided that women in this age group might not need mammograms. This flies in the face of what we know."
February 4, 1997	U.S. Senator Snowe	"Women and their doctors look to the Nation's preeminent cancer research institute—the National Cancer Institute—for clear guidance and advice on this issue. . . . By rescinding its guideline, NCI produced widespread confusion and concern among women and physicians regarding the appropriate age at which to seek mammograms."
February 4, 1997	US Senate Resolution 47	". . . we say enough is enough. We should take time out, go back to our science, go back to our research, go back to the National Institutes of Health and ask them to come up with the recommendation that we need."
March 27, 1997	National Cancer Institute	"The NCI advises women age 40–49 who are of average risk of breast cancer to have screening mammograms every year or two."

of disease in the total population is a result of the exposure?" the *population attributable risk* (PAR) is used. The PAR is calculated as follows:

$$\frac{P_e \,(\text{relative risk}_a - 1)}{1 + P_e \,(\text{relative risk}_a - 1)}$$

where P_e represents the proportion of the population that is exposed. Assuming that the relative risk$_a$ of lung cancer due to cigarette smoking is 15 (i.e., smokers have 15 times the risk of lung cancer compared with nonsmokers) and that 30% of the population are smokers, the population attributable risk is 0.81 or 81%. This would suggest that 81% of the lung cancer burden in the population is

Table 2–5. Modifiable Risk Factors for Coronary Heart Disease, United States

Magnitude	Risk Factor	Best Estimate (%) of Population Attributable Risk (Range)
Strong (relative risk >4)	None	—
Moderate (relative risk 2–4)	High blood pressure (≥140/90 mm Hg)	25 (20–29)
	Cigarette smoking	22 (17–25)
	Elevated cholesterol (≥200 mg/dL)	43 (39–47)
	Diabetes (fasting glucose ≥140 mg/dL)	8 (1–15)
Weak (relative risk <2)	Obesity[a]	17 (7–32)
	Physical inactivity	35 (23–46)
	Environmental tobacco smoke exposure	18 (8–23)
Possible	Psychological factors	—
	Alcohol use[b]	—
	Elevated plasma homocysteine	—
	Infectious agents	—

Source: From Newschaffer et al.[25]

[a]Based on body mass index >27.8 kg/m² for men and >27.3 kg/m² for women.

[b]Moderate to heavy alcohol use may increase risk, whereas light use may reduce risk.

caused by cigarette smoking and could be eliminated if the exposure were eliminated. Table 2–5 describes a variety of risk factors for coronary heart disease.[25] This list demonstrates that the greatest population burden (PAR) would be affected by eliminating elevated cholesterol and physical inactivity, even though the relative risk values for these risk factors are in the moderate or weak range.

A related metric is the prevented fraction (PF). In an intervention in which "exposure" to a program or policy may protect against disease, the PF is the proportion of disease occurrence in a population averted due to a protective risk factor or public health intervention.[26] The PF is calculated as follows:

$$P_e \text{ (relative risk}_b - 1)$$

where P_e represents the prevalence of exposure to the protective factor and relative risk$_b$ is a protective effect estimate (i.e., exposure to the preventive measure protects against acquiring a specific health problem). This formula for the PF is the same one used to calculate vaccine efficacy and has also been used to estimate the benefits of disease screening programs.[27]

Assessing Time Trends

There are numerous other factors that may be considered when weighing the need for public health action. One important factor to consider involves temporal

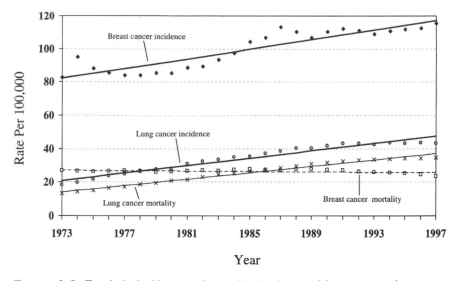

FIGURE 2–3. Trends in incidence and mortality for lung and breast cancer in women, United States, 1973–1997 (*Source*: Ries et al., 2000[28]).

trends (see chapter 5). Public health surveillance systems can provide information on changes over time in a risk factor or disease of interest. Through use of these data, one may determine whether the condition of interest is increasing, decreasing, or remaining constant. One may also examine the incidence or prevalence of a condition in relation to other conditions of interest. For example, if a public health practitioner were working with a statewide coalition to control cancer, it would be useful to plot both the incidence and mortality rates for various cancer sites (Figure 2–3).[28] The researcher might reach different conclusions on the impact and changing magnitude of various cancers when examining incidence versus mortality rates across the state. When working at a local level, however, it would be important to note that sample sizes might be too small for many health conditions, making rates unstable and subject to considerable fluctuations over time. In addition, a formal time-series analysis requires numerous data points (approximately 50 for the most sophisticated statistical methods). A simple and often useful time-series analysis can often be conducted with ordinary least-squares regression techniques, which are amenable to fewer data points than formal time-series analyses.

Priority Setting via National Health Goals

Determining public health and health care priorities in a climate of limited resources is a demanding task. In some cases, priority setting from experts and governmental bodies can help to focus areas for public health action. These efforts are particularly useful in evaluating Type I evidence (i.e., something must be done on a particular health topic). They are often less helpful for Type II evidence (i.e., this specific intervention should be conducted within a local area).

Public health leaders began to formulate concrete public health objectives as a basis for action during the post–World War II era. This was a clear shift from earlier efforts as emphasis was placed on quantifiable objectives and explicit time limits.[29] A few key examples illustrate the use of public data in setting and measuring progress toward health objectives. A paper by the Institute of Medicine[30] sparked a U.S. movement to set objectives for public health.[29] These initial actions by the Institute of Medicine led to the 1979 Surgeon General's Report on Health Promotion and Disease Prevention, which set five national goals—one each for the principal life stages of infancy, childhood, adolescence and young adulthood, adulthood, and older adulthood.[31]

More recently, the U.S. Public Health Service established two overarching health goals for the year 2010: (1) increase quality and years of healthy life; and (2) eliminate health disparities.[32] To achieve these two goals, a comprehensive set of objectives was established in twenty-eight focus areas. In support of these efforts, *Healthy People 2010* has also identified ten leading health indicators that will be used to set priorities and to measure the health of the United States over the next ten years (Table 2–6). The leading health indicators were selected on the basis of their ability to motivate action, the availability of data to measure progress, and their importance as public health issues.[32] In its earlier version *Healthy People 2000*), progress toward meeting objectives was measured in annual reports. Establishment of national, quantifiable objectives has stimulated state and local efforts in program and organizational planning. For example, an estimated 70% of all U.S. local health agencies (from a total of about 3,000) have used *Healthy People 2000* objectives.[33]

Table 2–6. Leading Health Indicators from *Healthy People 2010*

1. Physical Activity
2. Overweight and Obesity
3. Tobacco Use
4. Substance Abuse
5. Responsible Sexual Behavior
6. Mental Health
7. Injury and Violence
8. Environmental Quality
9. Immunization
10. Access to Health Care

SUMMARY

The issues covered in this chapter highlight one of the continuing challenges for public health practitioners and policy makers—determining when scientific evidence is sufficient for public health action. In nearly all instances, scientific studies cannot demonstrate causality with absolute certainty.[16, 34] The demarcation between action and inaction is seldom distinct and requires careful consideration of scientific evidence as well as assessment of values, preferences, costs, and benefits of various options. The difficulty in determining scientific certainty was eloquently summarized by A.B. Hill:[16]

All scientific work is incomplete—whether it be observational or experimental.
All scientific work is liable to be upset or modified by advancing knowledge.
That does not confer upon us a freedom to ignore the knowledge we already have, or to postpone the action that it appears to demand at a given time.

In many instances, waiting for absolute scientific certainty would mean delaying crucial public health action. For example, gaining a full understanding of the molecular biology of HIV/AIDS transmission prior to implementing population-based programs would have delayed important advances in prevention. Strong skills are crucial in understanding causality, interpreting the ever-expanding scientific literature, and seeking out summaries of evidence.

Other key points in this chapter:

- When considering public health action, it is helpful to consider the consequences of taking action or no action.
- Advances in epidemiology and public health research are generally incremental, suggesting the need for intervention as a body of literature accumulates.
- When evaluating literature, both the quality of component studies and their generalizability (external validity) should be considered.
- A set of standardized criteria can be useful in assessing the causality of an association.
- Many factors beyond science, such as resource constraints, sources of information, timing, and politics, influence decision-making in public health.

SUGGESTED READINGS AND WEBSITES

Readings

Briss PA, Zaza S, Pappaioanou M, et al. Developing an evidence-based Guide to Community Preventive Services—methods. The Task Force on Community Preventive Services. *American Journal of Preventive Medicine* 2000;18(1 Suppl):35–43.

Rothman KJ. Causes. *American Journal of Epidemiology* 1976;104:587–592.

Savitz DA, Harris RP, Brownson RC. Methods in chronic disease epidemiology. In: Brownson RC, Remington PL, Davis JR, eds. *Chronic Disease Epidemiology and Control.* 2nd ed. ed. Washington, DC: American Public Health Association, 1998, pp. 27–54.

Weed DL. On the use of causal criteria. *International Journal of Epidemiology* 1997; 26(6):1137–1141.

Selected Websites

Partners in Information Access for Public Health Professionals <http://www.nnlm.nlm. nih.gov/partners/>. A collaborative project to provide public health professionals with timely, convenient access to information resources to help them improve the health of the American public.

The Research Methods Knowledge Base <http://trochim.human.cornell.edu/kb/>. The Research Methods Knowledge Base is a comprehensive web-based textbook that addresses all of the topics in a typical introductory undergraduate or graduate course in social research methods. It covers the entire research process including: formulating research questions; sampling (probability and nonprobability); measurement (surveys, scaling, qualitative, unobtrusive); research design (experimental and quasi-experimental); data analysis; and, writing the research paper. It uses an informal, conversational style to engage both the newcomer and the more experienced student of research.

UCSF School of Medicine: Virtual Library in Epidemiology <http://chanane.ucsf. edu/epidem/> Large listing of websites in epidemiology and related fields is provided. Among the categories are governmental agencies, quantitative epidemiology, data sources, publications, and university sites.

REFERENCES

1. Savitz DA, Harris RP, Brownson RC. Methods in chronic disease epidemiology. In: Brownson RC, Remington PL and Davis JR, eds. *Chronic Disease Epidemiology and Control.* 2nd ed. Washington, DC: American Public Health Association, 1998, pp. 27–54.

2. U.S. Dept. of Health and Human Services. *Interim Report of the Long Island Breast Cancer Study Project.* Bethesda, MD: National Institutes of Health, June 2000.

3. Last JM, ed. *A Dictionary of Epidemiology.* 4th ed. New York: Oxford University Press, 2001.

4. Friis RH, Sellers TA. *Epidemiology for Public Health Practice.* 2nd ed. Gaithersburg, MD: Aspen Publishers, Inc., 1999.

5. Guyatt G, Rennie D, eds. *Users' Guides to the Medical Literature. A Manual for Evidence-Based Clinical Practice.* Chicago: American Medical Association Press, 2002.

6. Petitti DB. *Meta-analysis, Decision Analysis, and Cost-Effectiveness Analysis: Methods for Quantitative Synthesis in Medicine.* 2nd ed. New York: Oxford University Press, 2000.

7. Nelson DE. Assessing the science, locating information, and translating data. In: Nelson DE, Brownson RC, Remington PL, Parvanta C, eds. *Communicating Public Health Information Effectively: A Guide for Public Health Practitioners*. Washington, DC: American Public Health Association, (in press).

8. Briss PA, Zaza S, Pappaioanou M, et al. Developing an evidence-based Guide to Community Preventive Services—methods. The Task Force on Community Preventive Services. *American Journal of Preventive Medicine* 2000;18(1 Suppl):35–43.

9. Concato J, Shah N, Horwitz RI. Randomized, controlled trials, observational studies, and the hierachy of research designs. *New England Journal of Medicine* 2000;342: 1887–1892.

10. Beaglehole R, Bonita R, Kjellstrom T. *Basic Epidemiology*. Geneva, Switzerland: World Health Organization, 1993.

11. Pappaioanou M, Evans C. Developing a guide to community preventive services: A U.S. Public Health Service initiative. *Journal of Public Health Management and Practice*. 1998;4:48–54.

12. Truman BI, Smith-Akin CK, Hinman AR, et al. Developing the guide to community preventive services—overview and rationale. *American Journal of Preventive Medicine* 2000;18(1S):18–26.

13. Rivers TM. Viruses and Koch's postulates. *Journal of Bacteriology* 1937;33:1–12.

14. McKenna MT, Taylor WR, Marks JS, Koplan JP. Current issues and challenges in chronic disease control. In: Brownson RC, Remington PL and Davis JR, eds. *Chronic Disease Epidemiology and Control*. 2nd ed. Washington, DC: American Public Health Association; 1998 pp. 1–26.

15. U.S. Dept. of Health, Education, and Welfare,. *Smoking and Health. Report of the Advisory Committee to the Surgeon General of the Public Health Service*. Vol. Publication (PHS) 1103. Washington, DC: Center for Disease Control, 1964.

16. Hill AB. The environment and disease: association or causation? *Proceedings of the Royal Society of Medicine* 1965;58:295–300.

17. Susser M. *Causal Thinking in the Health Sciences: Concepts and Strategies in Epidemiology*. New York: Oxford University Press, 1973.

18. Rothman KJ. Causes. *American Journal of Epidemiology* 1976;104:587–592.

19. Kelsey JL. *Methods in Observational Epidemiology*. 2nd ed. New York: Oxford University Press, 1996.

20. Weed DL. Epidemiologic evidence and causal inference. *Hematology/Oncology Clinics of North America* 2000;14(4):797–807.

21. Weed DL. On the use of causal criteria. *International Journal of Epidemiology* 1997; 26(6):1137–1141.

22. Bero LA, Jadad AR. How consumers and policy makers can use systematic reviews for decision making. In: Mulrow C, Cook D, eds. *Systematic Reviews. Synthesis of Best Evidence for Health Care Decisions*. Philadelphia: American College of Physicians, 1998, pp. 45–54.

23. U.S. Preventive Services Task Force. *Guide to Clinical Preventive Services*. 2nd ed. Baltimore: Williams & Wilkins, 1996.

24. Ernster VL. Mammography screening for women aged 40 through 49—A guidelines saga and a clarion call for informed decision making. *American Journal of Public Health* 1997;87(7):1103–1106.

25. Newschaffer CJ, Brownson CA, Dusenbury LJ. Cardiovascular disease. In: Brownson RC, Remington PL and Davis JR, eds. *Chronic Disease Epidemiology and Con-*

trol. 2nd ed. Washington, DC: American Public Health Association, 1998, pp. 297–334.

26. Gargiullo PM, Rothenberg RB, Wilson HG. Confidence intervals, hypothesis tests, and sample sizes for the prevented fraction in cross-sectional studies. *Statistics in Medicine* 1995;14(1):51–72.

27. Straatman H, Verbeek AL, Peeters PH. Etiologic and prevented fraction in case-control studies of screening. *Journal of Clinical Epidemiology.* 1988;41(8):807–811.

28. Ries LAG, Eisner MP, Kosary CL, et al., eds. *SEER Cancer Statistics Review, 1973–1997.* Bethesda, MD: National Cancer Institute, 2000.

29. Breslow L. The future of public health: Prospects in the United States for the 1990s. *Annual Review of Public Health* 1990;11:1–28.

30. Nightingale EO, Cureton M, Kamar V, Trudeau MB. *Perspectives on Health Promotion and Disease Prevention in the United States.* [staff paper]. Washington, DC: Institute of Medicine, National Academy of Sciences, 1978.

31. U.S. Dept. of Health Education, and Welfare. *Healthy People. The Surgeon General's Report on Health Promotion and Disease Prevention.* Washington, DC: U.S. Dept. of Health, Education, and Welfare, 1979. Publication no. 79–55071.

32. U.S. Dept. of Health and Human Services. *Healthy People 2010. Volume II. Conference Edition.* Washington, DC: U.S. Dept. of Health and Human Services, 2000.

33. National Association of County and City Health Officials. *1992–1993 National Profile of Local Health Departments. National Surveillance Series.* Washington, DC. National Association of County and City Health Officials, 1995.

34. Susser M. Judgement and causal inference: Criteria in epidemiologic studies. *American Journal of Epidemiology* 1977;105:1–15.

35. Centers for Disease Control. Toxic-shock syndrome—United States. *Morbidity and Mortality Weekly Report* 1980;29:229–230.

36. Shands KN, Schmid GP, Dan BB, et al. Toxic-shock syndrome in menstruating women: Association with tampon use and Staphylococcus aureus and clinical features in 52 cases. *New England Journal of Medicine* 1980;303:1436–1442.

37. Schuchat A, Broome CV. Toxic shock syndrome and tampons *Epidemiologic Reviews.* 1991;13:99–112.

38. American Cancer Society. *Cancer Facts & Figures 2000.* Atlanta: American Cancer Society, 2000. 00–300M-No. 5008.00.

39. Breslow L, et al. Final Report of NCI Ad Hoc Working Groups on Mammography in Screening for Breast Cancer. *Journal of the National Cancer Institute* 1977;59(2):469–541.

40. American Cancer Society. Report on the Cancer-Related Health Checkup. *CA: A Cancer Journal of Clinicians* 1980;30:193–196.

41. National Institutes of Health Consensus Development Panel. National Institutes of Health Consensus Development Conference Statement: Breast Cancer Screening for Women Ages 40–49, January 21–23, 1997. *Journal of the National Cancer Institute* 1997;89:1015–1026.

3

Understanding and Applying
Analytic Tools

> There are in fact two things: science and opinion. One begets
> knowledge, the latter ignorance.
>
> —Hippocrates

The preceding chapters have underlined the desirability of using evidence to
inform decision making in public health. The first chapter gave an overview and
definitions of evidence-based practice. The second chapter described the scientific factors to consider when determining whether some type of public health
action is warranted. This chapter describes several useful tools for evidence-
based public health practice, such as systematic reviews and economic evaluation, that help practitioners answer the question, "Is this program or policy worth
doing?"

Chapter 3 has five main parts. First, we describe some context and processes
for developing systematic reviews and economic evaluations. Then we discuss
several analytic tools for measuring risk and intervention effectiveness (e.g.,
systematic reviews, meta-analysis). The third part describes comparative tools
for comparing benefits and costs. One particular type of economic evaluation,
cost-utility analysis, is described in greater detail in this section. In the fourth
section, several challenges and opportunities in using these analytic tools are
discussed. The chapter concludes with a short discussion of processes for translating evidence into public health action (e.g., expert panels, practice guidelines).
A major goal of this chapter is to help readers develop an understanding of these
evidence-based methods and an appreciation of their usefulness. We seek to
assist practitioners in becoming informed users of various analytic tools for
decision making. The chapter does not provide detailed descriptions of the mechanics of conducting various types of analytic reviews—readers are referred to
several excellent sources for these elements.[1–5]

BACKGROUND

A review can be thought of as a more comprehensive, modern-day equivalent of the encyclopedia article. Traditionally, an encyclopedia article was written by a person knowledgeable in a subject area, who was charged with reviewing the literature and writing a summary assessment of the current state of the art on that particular topic.

A systematic review uses a formal approach to identify and synthesize the existing knowledge base and prespecifies key questions of interest in an attempt to find all of the relevant literature addressing those questions. It also systematically assesses the quality of identified papers. Systematic reviews can address any number of problems and have recently been used in advertising, astronomy, criminology, ecology, entomology, and parapsychology.[6] In this chapter, we will focus our discussion on reviews of the effectiveness of interventions to improve health. The goal of a systematic review is an unbiased assessment of a particular topic, such as interventions to improve vaccination rates or to reduce smoking rates, that summarizes a large amount of information, identifies beneficial or harmful interventions, and points out gaps in the scientific literature.[7] Systematic reviews can be conducted in many ways—by an individual, a small team of researchers, or a larger expert panel. It is sometimes stipulated that such a review include a quantitative synthesis (i.e., meta-analysis) of the data.[8] In this chapter, however, the outcome of the systematic review process is defined as a narrative (qualitative) assessment of the literature, a practice guideline, or a quantitative statistical combination of results like a meta-analysis.

Economic evaluation aims at improving the allocation of scarce resources. Given that we cannot afford to do everything, how do we choose among projects? Economic evaluation identifies and weighs the relative costs and benefits of competing alternatives so that the project with the least costs for a given benefit, or the greatest benefits for a given cost, should be chosen. Like systematic reviews, economic evaluations can use the existing literature to forecast the impact of a proposed program or policy. However, economic evaluations can also use prospective data to determine the cost-effectiveness of a new project. As a result, economic evaluations are increasingly being conducted alongside clinical trials.[9, 10] The essential difference between the two methods is their aim. Systematic reviews can cover any of a broad array of topics, such as the epidemiology of a particular disease or condition, the effectiveness of an intervention, or the economic costs of a particular treatment. Economic evaluations have a narrower focus and deal primarily with costs and benefits: What benefits will be gained at what cost?

TOOLS FOR ASSESSING RISK AND INTERVENTION EFFECTIVENESS

A number of analytic tools are available to assess risk of exposure to a particular factor (e.g., cigarette smoking, lack of mammography screening). Other tools are focused less on etiologic research and more on measuring the effectiveness of a particular public health intervention. To provide an overview of several useful tools, we will describe systematic reviews, meta-analysis, pooled analysis, and risk assessment.

Systematic Reviews

As noted earlier, systematic reviews are syntheses of comprehensive collections of information on a particular topic. Reading a good review can be one of the most efficient ways to become familiar with state-of-the-art research and practice on many specific topics in public health.[11-14] The use of explicit, systematic methods in reviews limits bias and reduces chance effects, thus providing more reliable results upon which to make decisions.[15] Numerous approaches are used in developing systematic reviews. All systematic reviews have important common threads as well as important differences but this chapter focuses primarily on the similarities. General methods used in a systematic review as well as several types of reviews and their practical applications are described below. More detailed descriptions of these methods are available in the *JAMA Users' Guides to the Medical Literature*[16] and Mulrow and Cook.[17] Several authors have provided checklists that can be useful in assessing the methodologic quality of a systematic review article (Table 3-1).[16, 18, 19]

Methods for Conducting a Systematic Review.   The goal of this section is not to teach readers how to conduct a systematic review but to provide a basic understanding of the six common steps in conducting a systematic review. Each is briefly summarized and some selected differences in approaches are discussed.

Identify the problem.   The first step in a systematic review is the identification of the problem. Reviewing the literature, considering the practical aspects of the problem, and talking to experts in the area are all ways to begin to develop a concise statement of the problem (see Chapter 4). Systematic reviews focusing on effectiveness typically begin with a formal statement of the issue to be addressed. This usually includes statements of the intervention under study, the population in which it might be used, the outcomes being considered, and the relevant comparison. For example, the problem might be to determine the effectiveness of screening for Type II diabetes in adult African American men to

Table 3–1. Checklist for Evaluating the Methodologic Quality of a Systematic Review

Are the results valid?
• Did the review explicitly address a focused and answerable question?
• Based on the search process, is it likely that important, relevant studies were missed?
• Were the primary studies of high methodologic quality?
• Were assessments of studies reproducible?

What are the results?
• Were the results similar from study to study?
• How precise were the results?
• Do the pooled results allow you to examine subgroup differences?
• Can a causal association be inferred from the available data?

How can I apply the results to patient care and/or population health?
• How can I best interpret the results to apply them to the care of patients in my practice or populations that I serve in my public health agency?
• Were all outcomes of clinical and public health importance considered?
• Are the benefits worth the costs and potential risks?

Source: adapted from Kelsey et al.,[18] Oxman et al.,[19] Guyatt and Rennie.[16]

reduce the occurrence of macrovascular and microvascular complications of diabetes compared to usual care. Problem identification should also include a description of where the information for the systematic review will be obtained, e.g., information will come from a search of the literature over the last ten years.

Search the literature.   There are numerous electronic databases available, and one or more of these should be systematically searched. Several of these are excellent sources of published literature as well. These databases and the method for literature searching are described in detail in Chapter 6. For a variety of reasons, however, limiting searching to electronic databases can have drawbacks:

• Most systematic reviews use the published literature as the source of their data. Databases, however, may not include technical or final reports. If these are thought to be important relative to the intervention being considered, then a source for these documents should be identified and searched.
• Published studies may be subject to publication bias—the tendency of research with statistically significant results to be submitted and published over results that are not statistically significant and/or null.[4] To reduce the likelihood of publication bias, some reviews go to considerable lengths to find additional unpublished studies. (See Chapter 2, section on publication bias).
• Even the best database searches typically find only one-half to two-thirds of the available literature. Reviews of reference lists and consultations with experts are very helpful in finding additional sources. Often, advice from experts

in the field, national organizations, and governmental public health agencies can be very helpful.

Apply inclusion and exclusion criteria.   The third step is to develop inclusion and exclusion criteria for those studies to be reviewed. This step often leads to revision and further specification of the problem statement. Common issues include the study design, the level of analysis, the type of analysis, and the source(s) and time frame for study retrieval. The inclusion and exclusion criteria should be selected so as to yield those studies most relevant to the purpose of the systematic review. If the purpose of the systematic review is to assess the effectiveness of interventions to increase physical activity rates among school children, for example, then interventions aimed at representative populations (e.g., those including adults) would be excluded. Ideally as the inclusion and exclusion criteria are applied, at least a portion of the data retrieval should be repeated by a second person, and results should be compared. If discrepancies are found, the inclusion and exclusion criteria are probably not sufficiently specific or clear. They should be reviewed and revised as needed.

Study design.   The first issue to consider is the type of study. Should only randomized controlled trials be included? Some would answer "yes" because randomized controlled trials are said to provide the most reliable data and to be specially suited for supporting causal inference. Others would argue that randomized controlled trials also have their limitations, such as contamination or questionable external validity, and that including a broader range of designs could increase the aggregate internal and external validity of the entire body of evidence. An additional problem with limiting public health systematic reviews to randomized trials is that there are many public health areas in which this would result in no studies being possible (because trials would be unethical or infeasible). Observational and quasi-experimental studies are appropriate designs for many intervention topics. There may also be characteristics of a study that are necessary for inclusion, such as that baseline and follow-up assessment he made in conjunction with the intervention and/or that a comparison group he used.

Level of analysis.   The inclusion and exclusion criteria for level of analysis should match the purpose of the systematic review. The most salient feature for public health is whether studies are at the individual or the community level. A potentially confusing problem, especially if one is interested in assessing community-based interventions, is what to do with "mixed" studies—those that include interventions aimed at both the community and the individual. A good strategy in that case is to include all related studies in the data searching and then use the data abstraction form (described below) to determine whether the study should remain in the data set.

Type of analysis. Evaluations of interventions can use several methods. Some, like the use of focus groups, are more qualitative; others, such as regression modeling, are more quantitative. Often, the specification of the question will make some types of studies relevant and others off-topic. Some questions can be addressed in varied ways, and when this is true, broad inclusiveness might give more complete answers. However, the more disparate the methodologies included, the more difficult it is to combine and consolidate the results. A qualitative approach to the review tends to be more inclusive, collecting information from all types of analysis. Meta-analysis, because it consolidates results using a statistical methodology, requires quantitative analysis.

Data sources and time frame. The final items to be specified are where a search for studies will be conducted and the time period to be covered. The natural history of the intervention should help determine the time frame. A major change in the delivery of an intervention, for example, makes it difficult to compare results from studies before and after the new delivery method. In this case, one might limit the time to the "after" period. An additional factor influencing time frame is the likely applicability of the results. Sometimes, substantial changes in context have occurred over time. For example, results from the 1960s may be of questionable relevance to the current situation. In that case, one might limit the review to more recent data. A pragmatic factor influencing the selection of a time frame is the availability of electronic databases.

Conduct data abstraction.   Once the inclusion and exclusion criteria have been specified, the next step is to find the studies that fit your framework, and then to extract a common set of information from them. In general, a data abstraction form should be used. This form should direct the systematic extraction of key information about the elements of the study so that they can be consolidated and assessed. Typical elements include the number of participants, the type of study, a precise description of the intervention, and the results for the study. If the data abstraction form is well designed, the data consolidation and assessment can proceed, using only the forms. The exact format and content of the abstraction form depends upon the intervention and the type of analysis being used in the systematic review. An excellent and comprehensive example of an abstraction form is provided by the Task Force on Community Preventive Services.[5]

Consolidate the evidence.   The next step in a systematic review is an assessment of whether data from the various studies can be combined. (Often they should not if, for example, all of the available studies have serious flaws or if the interventions or outcomes are too disparate.) If data can be combined to reach an overall conclusion, it may be done either qualitatively or quantitatively.

Assessment and conclusion.   Once the evidence has been consolidated, the final step is to assess it and reach a conclusion. For example, suppose that the intervention being reviewed is the launching of mass media campaigns to increase physical activity rates among adults. Further, assume that a meta-analysis of this topic reveals that a majority of studies find that community-based interventions improve physical activity rates. However, the effect size is small. What should the review conclude?

The review must consider both the strength and weight of the evidence and the substantive importance of the effect. This assessment can be done by the reviewer using his or her own internal criteria, or by using explicit criteria that were set before the review was conducted. An example of the latter approach is the method employed by the U.S. Preventive Services Task Force (USPSTF).[20] The USPSTF looks at the quality and weight of the evidence (rated Good, Fair, or Poor), and the net benefit, or effect size, of the preventive service (rated Substantial, Moderate, Small, and Zero/negative). Their overall rating and recommendation reflects a combination of these two factors. For example, if a systematic review of a preventive service finds "Fair" evidence of a "Substantial" effect, the Task Force gives it a recommendation of "B," or a recommendation that clinicians routinely provide the service to eligible patients.

If no formal process for combining the weight of the evidence and the substantive importance of the findings has been specified beforehand, and the systematic review yields mixed findings, then it is useful to seek help with assessing the evidence and drawing a conclusion. The analyst might ask experts in the field to review the evidence and reach a conclusion or make a recommendation.

After completing the systematic review, the final step is to write up a report and disseminate the findings. The report should include a description of all of the above steps. Ideally, the systematic review should be disseminated to the potential users of the recommendations. The method of dissemination should be targeted to the desired audience. Increasingly, this means putting reports on the Internet so that they are freely accessible or presenting the findings to a community planning board. However, it is also important to submit reviews for publication in peer-reviewed journals. This provides one final quality check. Various methods for disseminating the results of systematic reviews are described later in this chapter.

Meta-Analysis

Over the past two decades, meta-analysis has been increasingly used to synthesize the findings of multiple research studies. Meta-analysis was originally developed in the social sciences in the 1970s when hundreds of studies existed on the same topics.[4] The key contribution of meta-analysis has been to provide a systematic, replicable, and objective method of integrating the findings of individual studies.[21] Meta-analysis uses a quantitative approach to summarize evidence, in which results from separate studies are pooled to obtain a weighted average summary result.[4, 22] Its use has appeal because of its potential to pool a group of smaller studies, enhancing statistical power. It also may allow reseachers to test subgroup effects (e.g., by gender or age group) that are sometimes difficult to assess in a single, smaller study. Suppose there were several studies examining the effects of exercise on cholesterol levels, with each reporting the average change in cholesterol levels, the standard deviation of that change, and the number of study participants. These average changes could be weighted by sample size and pooled to obtain an average of the averages[23] change in cholesterol levels. If this grand mean showed a significant decline in cholesterol levels among exercisers, then the meta-analyst would conclude that the evidence supported exercise as a way to lower cholesterol levels. Box 3–1 describes a recent meta-analysis of the relationship between alcohol consumption and breast cancer.[24]

Similar to the method described above for conducting a systematic review, Petitti notes four essential steps in conducting a meta-analysis: (1) identifying relevant studies; (2) deciding upon inclusion and exclusion criteria for studies under consideration; (3) abstracting the data; and 4) conducting the statistical analysis, including exploration of heterogeneity.[4]

Meta-analysis includes several different statistical methods for aggregating the results from multiple studies. The method chosen depends on the type of analysis used in the original studies, which, in turn, is related to the type of data analyzed. For example, continuous data, such as cholesterol levels, can be analyzed by comparing the means of different groups. Continuous data could also be analyzed with multiple linear regression. Discrete (dichotomous) data are often analyzed with relative risks or odds ratios, although a range of other options also exists.

An important issue for meta-analysis is the similarity of studies to be combined. This similarity, or homogeneity, is assessed using various statistical tests. If studies are too dissimilar (high heterogeneity), then combining their results is problematic. One approach is to combine only homogenous subsets of studies. While statistically appealing, this to some extent defeats the purpose of the systematic review because a single summary assessment of the evidence is not reported. An alternative approach is to use meta-analytic methods that allow the addition of control variables that measure the differences among studies. For example, studies may differ by type of study design. If so, then a new variable could be created to code different study design types, such as observational and randomized controlled trials.

The statistical issue of the similarity of studies is related to the inclusion and

Box 3–1. Meta-Analysis of the Effect of Alcohol Consumption on the Risk of Breast Cancer

The relationship between alcohol consumption and the risk of breast cancer has been examined in numerous studies over the years. After all of these studies, what can we conclude? Does alcohol consumption increase the risk of breast cancer? A recent meta-analysis found that the answer to this question is a mild "yes": alcohol use increases the risk of breast cancer, but by a small amount.[24]

To arrive at this answer, the authors searched MEDLINE, an electronic database, from 1966 to 1999 for studies of the relationship between alcohol consumption and breast cancer. They then looked at the references cited in these articles to find additional articles. This approach identified seventy-four publications. Next, they reviewed the publications to see if they met the inclusion and exclusion criteria they had specified. Inclusion criteria included such requirements as reporting alcohol intake in a manner that could be converted to grams of alcohol per day and reporting data from an original cohort or case-control study. Exclusion criteria included items such as reports that were published only as letters to the editor or abstracts and studies that had implausible results. After applying the inclusion and exclusion criteria, forty-two reports remained.

These forty-two reports were then carefully reviewed and abstracted. The number of participants, alcohol consumption, incidence of breast cancer, and presence of several confounders for the group were extracted from each study. The authors used regression analysis to combine the aggregate data from the various studies and estimate a dose-response relationship between alcohol consumption and breast cancer risk. Using regression analysis also allowed them to control for and examine the effects of various confounders, such as study site (hospital-based or other) and type of alcoholic beverage. In comparison with nondrinkers, women consuming an average of 6 grams of alcohol per day (approximately one-half of a typical alcoholic drink) had a 4.9 percent increased risk of breast cancer (95 % confidence interval (CI) 1.03–1.07). Women consuming one (12 grams of alcohol) or two (24 grams of alcohol) drinks per day had increased risks of 10% (95% CI 1.06–1.14) and 21% (95% CI 1.13–1.30), respectively.

exclusion criteria. These criteria are selected to identify a group of studies for review that are similar in a substantive way. If the meta-analysis finds that the studies are not statistically homogeneous, then the source of heterogeneity should be investigated. This part of the meta-analysis thus forces a reconsideration of the inclusion and exclusion criteria.[25] A careful search for the sources of heterogeneity and a consideration of their substantive importance can improve the overall systematic review.

Meta-analysis has generated a fair amount of controversy, particularly when it is used to combine results of observational studies.[4, 18, 26] The quality of the meta-analysis depends heavily on the explicit delineation of the criteria for selection of the specific studies eligible for inclusion in the meta-analysis. Journal articles based on meta-analysis need to be read in the same critical manner as articles based on original research. Despite its limitations, a properly done meta-analysis provides a rigorous way of integrating the findings of several studies. Because it follows a set of specified guidelines, it can be less subjective than the usual qualitative review that weights and combines studies, based upon the expert opinion of the authors.[18]

Pooled Analysis

Unlike meta-analysis, which uses data aggregated at the study level, pooled analysis refers to the analysis of data from multiple studies at the level of the individual participant. The goals of a pooled analysis are the same as a meta-analysis, i.e., obtaining a quantitative estimate of effect.[4] This type of systematic review is much less common than others described in this chapter and has received less formal treatment in the literature. Nonetheless, it has proved informative in characterizing dose-response relationships for certain environmental risks that may be etiologically related to a variety of chronic diseases. For example, pooled analyses on radiation risks have been published for nuclear workers,[27] underground miners,[28] and for women who received repeated fluoroscopy in the management of tuberculosis.[29]

Risk Assessment

Quantitative risk assessment is a widely used term for a systematic approach to characterizing the risks posed to individuals and populations by environmental pollutants and other potentially adverse exposures.[30, 31] Risk assessment has been described as a "bridge" between science and policy making.[32] In the United States, its use is either explicitly or implicitly required by a number of federal statutes, and its application worldwide is increasing. Risk assessment has become an established process through which expert scientific input is provided to agencies that regulate environmental or occupational exposures. Four key steps in risk assessment are hazard identification, risk characterization, exposure assessment, and risk estimation.[31] An important aspect of risk assessment is that it frequently results in classification schemes that take into account uncertainties about exposure–disease relationships. For example, the U.S. Environmental Protection Agency (EPA) developed a five-tier scheme for classifying potential and proven cancer-causing agents that includes the following: (1) Group A—carcinogenic to humans, (2) Group B—probably carcinogenic to humans; (3) Group C—possibly carcinogenic to humans; (4) Group D—not classifiable as to human carcinogenicity; and (5) Group E—evidence of non-carcinogenicity for humans.[33]

TOOLS FOR COMPARING OPTIONS AND WEIGHING BENEFITS VERSUS COSTS

When comparing a variety of options for intervention, decision analysis and economic evaluation may be particularly useful.

Decision Analysis

Decision analysis is a derivative of operations research and game theory that involves the identification of all available choices and potential outcomes of each in a visual series of decisions.[34] Along with each choice in the "decision tree," probabilities of outcomes are estimated that arise at decision nodes. An example of a decision tree is shown in Figure 3–1. This tree is based upon a study of exercise to prevent coronary heart disease among males.[35] The study estimated what would happen to two hypothetical cohorts of one thousand 35-year-old

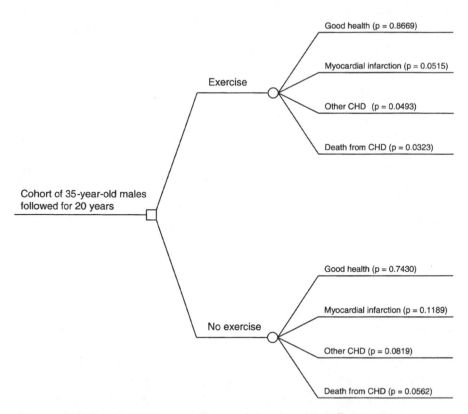

FIGURE 3–1. Sample decision tree for exercise to prevent cardiac events among men (based on data from Hatziandreu et al.[35]). CHD, coronary heart disease.

men over thirty years if one cohort jogged and the other did not. To estimate the effects of exercise, the authors had to identify all of the outcomes relevant to coronary heart disease (the branches of the tree) and use the literature to find the prevalence of these events over a thirty-year time span (the probabilities below the branches of the tree).

Decision analysis has historically been used to help inform complex decisions under conditions of uncertainty. It has been widely used by clinicians to make decisions about individual patients. Increasingly, decision analysis has been used to develop policies about the management of groups of patients by looking for the "best" outcome for the most value,[4] and is often a fundamental component of an economic evaluation.[36] In the latter case, the tree is modified to include the costs and benefits of each branch as well as the probabilities.

There are five steps in a decision analysis:[37]

1. Identifying and bounding the problem
2. Structuring the problem
3. Gathering information to fill the decision tree
4. Analyzing the decision tree
5. Harnessing uncertainty by conducting a sensitivity analysis

The first two steps help one to draw the decision tree. Step 3, "gathering information," can be done by using new data or by surveying the literature. For a standard decision tree, the probability of reaching each branch and the number of persons who will enter the tree are the two essential pieces of information. For an economic evaluation, the tree must also include the costs and benefits of each branch.

The decision tree is analyzed by starting a (hypothetical) number of persons at the base of the tree. Based on the probabilities found at each branching point, a certain number of persons go to different branches. The process stops when all of the persons have reached one of the far right-hand branches, which represent the final outcomes. For example, of the 1000 men who jog, 32 (1000 * 0.0323) will die from coronary heart disease (CHD) after thirty years, while 56 (1000 * 0.0562) of those who do not exercise will die from CHD. The numbers of people at the final outcomes of interest are then compared and a conclusion reached. Using Figure 3–1 and comparing the number of CHD-related deaths among exercisers and nonexercisers, one could conclude that exercise reduces the number of deaths by one-half.[35]

The fifth step is to conduct a sensitivity analysis. Decision analysis in medicine arose in part to reflect and analyze the uncertainty of treatment outcomes. The probability assigned to each branch is the average likelihood of that particular outcome. In practice, the actual probability may turn out to be higher or lower. Sensitivity analysis varies the probability estimates and reanalyzes the tree. The less the outcomes vary as the probabilities are altered, the more robust is the result. There are several ways to conduct a sensitivity analysis and this technique is discussed further in the context of economic evaluation later in this chapter.

Decision analysis is especially useful for a clinical or policy decision under the following conditions:[4, 38]

- The decision is complex and information is uncertain
- Viable choices exist that are legal, ethical, and not cost prohibitive
- The decision is a close call and consequences are important

Decision analysis can be informative because it forces the analyst to explicitly list all the potential outcomes and pathways and the likelihood of each. Often, the process itself is illuminating, especially if there are complex pathways involved.

Economic Evaluation

Economic evaluation is the comparison of costs and benefits to determine the most efficient allocation of scarce resources. We undertake economic evaluations all the time in everyday life, though we seldom think of the process explicitly. For example, ordering dinner at a restaurant requires weighing the costs (dollars and calories) versus the benefits (nutrition and flavor) of all of the options. Then, we choose an entrée that is the "best" use of our resources (dollars)—the best value for the money. This implicit weighing of costs and benefits is almost automatic, though we've probably all faced a menu that offered too many options at one time or another. In most public health applications, however, weighing the costs and benefits does not happen so automatically.

What are the distinguishing features of public health that require a formal economic evaluation? Consider three features of the restaurant example. First, the costs and benefits are all borne by one person, the diner, who has an incentive to compare costs and benefits and make a wise choice. Second, the information needed for the choice is fairly easy to obtain. The entrees are described on the menu, the prices are listed, and the diner knows his or her own palate and preferences. Finally, the stakes are fairly low. A bad decision can be remedied by sending the meal back to the kitchen or by avoiding the entrée or restaurant the next time the diner eats out.

All three of these characteristics are absent from most public health decisions. First, by their nature, public health programs are aimed at improving the health of a community, so benefits will be spread over a large number of people. Costs are also typically spread over a large group, often through taxation. Second, the information about costs and benefits may not be easy to obtain. Benefits and costs must be measured over many people. Often, the benefits include hard-to-measure items like improved health status. Third, the stakes are often relatively high. Programs may be expensive and resources scarce, so only a few of a large range of interventions may be funded. A bad choice cannot easily be remedied.

Types of Economic Evaluation.   There are four interrelated types of economic evaluation: cost–benefit analysis (CBA), cost-effectiveness analysis (CEA), cost-utility analysis (CUA), and cost-minimization analysis. This chapter explains CUA in greater detail; the other methods are then compared briefly to it. CUA is singled out because it is the recommended method of the U.S. Public Health Service Panel on Cost-Effectiveness Analysis[2] and because it is the most commonly used method today.

The four methods differ primarily in the way that they measure benefits. Cost-benefit analysis measures benefits in dollars, whereas CEA measures benefits in an appropriate health unit (e.g., lives saved). Cost-utility analysis is a type of CEA in which benefits (e.g., life years saved) are adjusted for the loss of quality of life and quantified with a health utility measure (usually quality-adjusted life years, or QALYs). Cost-minimization analysis is only used when the benefits of the two interventions are identical, so the unit of measurement of benefits is not an issue. Because CBA uses the most "generic" outcome measure (many things can be measured in dollars, including the value of transportation projects and educational interventions) it allows for the comparison of the most programs. As we move to CEA, then to CUA, and finally to cost-minimization analysis, the range of programs that can be compared narrows.

Outcomes of an Economic Evaluation.   Figure 3–2 shows the potential outcomes of an economic evaluation.[36] Consider the four quadrants of the graph. Programs that improve health and save money (Quadrant IV) are obviously worthwhile and should be undertaken. Similarly, programs that worsen health and add to costs (Quadrant II) are undesirable and should not be initiated or continued. The remaining two quadrants (I and III) are where the dilemmas lie and where economic evaluation can be informative.

Historically, as public health systems and nations develop, interventions and programs begin in Quadrant IV, with those programs that are both cost saving and improve health. Many early public health interventions, such as sanitation systems, fall in Quadrant IV. Once these interventions are exploited and implemented, attention turns to Quadrant I, programs that improve health at some

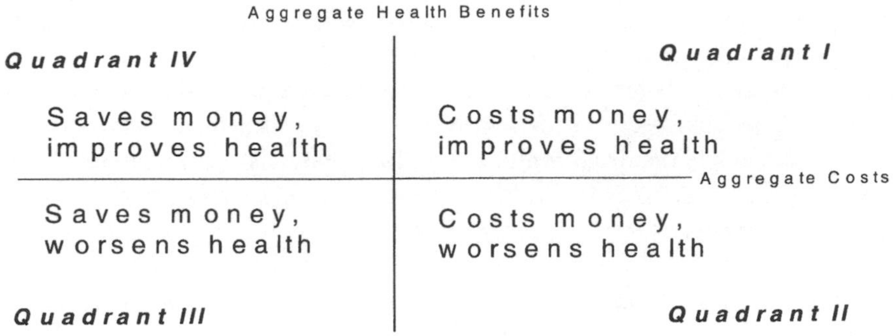

Aggregate Health Benefits

Quadrant IV	**Quadrant I**
Saves money, improves health	Costs money, improves health
	———— Aggregate Costs
Saves money, worsens health	Costs money, worsens health
Quadrant III	**Quadrant II**

FIGURE 3–2. Possible outcomes of an economic evaluation (adapted from Drummond et al.[36]).

cost. Eventually, as budgetary pressures increase, Quadrant III programs are considered: programs that reduce costs, but at some loss of health status. For both of these quadrants, the question is, what is the return on the investment (or disinvestment) of the public's funds? Economic evaluation provides a way to answer this question so that programs with the greatest return on investment can be selected.

Conceptual Framework for Economic Evaluation. In the above example, several key conceptual elements of economic evaluation can be identified. Before considering the mechanics of conducting an economic evaluation, it may be useful to determine the general elements and approach of all economic evaluations.

The first element is the selection of the perspective of the economic evaluation. Any intervention can be considered from several points of view, often characterized as moving from narrow to broad. The narrowest perspective is that of the agency or organization directly involved in delivering the proposed intervention. A next level might be the perspective of insurers, or payers, especially in health, where consumers and payers are often two separate groups. The broadest perspective is that of society as a whole. The U.S. Panel on Cost-Effectiveness in Health Care recommends this broad perspective for all economic evaluations.[2] This perspective is the most appropriate in public health because interventions are designed to benefit the public and taxpayers who fund the costs.

The next stage is the identification and measurement of all costs, including incremental costs of a program, option, or intervention. Incremental costs are the additional costs related to the program. If such costs are concentrated among a small group of people, this step will be relatively easy. As costs are more dispersed, it may become more difficult to identify all potential costs. Measurement of the identified costs may similarly be complicated by issues of units of measurement (e.g., dollar wages vs. donated labor time) and timing (e.g., costs incurred over a five year interval).

The third conceptual element is the identification and measurement of all benefits. Again, the incremental benefits are of interest: what additional benefits will this program provide, compared to some specified alternative? This step is often more complicated than the identification and measurement of costs. In public health, benefits can include improved health status (cases prevented) and improved mortality outcomes (deaths averted). Clearly, these benefits will be difficult to measure and will be partially subjective.

A fourth element is the comparison of costs and benefits. One can think of placing costs on one side of a balance, or scale, and benefits on the other. To which side does the scale tip? If the costs and benefits are measured in the same units (e.g., dollars) then this question is easy to answer. If, as is usually the case, the costs are in dollars and the benefits are in some health outcome measure, then it is difficult to see whether the balance is tipping towards the costs or the benefits side. Instead of placing costs and benefits on the two sides of a scale, the best assessment that can be made is that it costs X dollars per unit of health benefit. This is found by forming a ratio, with costs in the numerator and benefits in the denominator:

$$\text{Economic evaluation ratio} = \frac{\text{Incremental costs}}{\text{Incremental benefits}}$$

The final conceptual element is the interpretation of the results. If one finds, for example, that a program costs $27,000 per life saved, is the program worthwhile? There are numerous ways to approach this question, involving ethics, practical considerations, political realities, and economics. One could argue that, clearly, a life is worth $27,000, and the program is worthwhile. If, however, there is another program that costs $15,000 per life saved and the budget allows only one to be funded, an argument can be made that the latter program is more worthwhile than the former.

Determining costs.   The first step in an economic evaluation is to identify and determine all the costs of the intervention. These will be summed to form the numerator of the cost-utility (or cost-benefit or cost-effectiveness) ratio. Table 3–2 shows the types of costs and their usual measures. The labels and definitions for the types of costs vary across disciplines and across textbooks. The important objective of the cost portion of the analysis is the identification and determination of *all* costs, regardless of their labels.

The first category of costs is direct, or program, costs. One caution in stating

Table 3–2. Types of Costs Included in Economic Evaluations

Category of Cost	Usual Measures and Examples
Direct or Program Costs	
Labor	Wages and fringe benefits
Supplies	Supplies for the intervention, including office supplies, screening tests, materials
Overhead	Allocation for office space, rent, utilities
Indirect Costs	
Positive indirect costs; to be added to costs	
Time and travel costs	Time costs to participants, including lost wages
	Travel costs to participants, including transportation and child care
	Caregiver costs, including both time and travel
	Any costs of the program incurred by other budgetary groups
Cost of treating side effects	Cost of treatment; using actual cost or charge data or imputed, using local, regional, or national averages.
Cost of treatment during gained life expectancy	National data on average cost of treatment per year, multiplied by extended life expectancy
Negative indirect costs (benefits); to be subtracted from costs	
Averted treatment costs	Weighted sum of the cost of treatment, including alternative options and complications. Weights reflect the proportion of people projected to have each alternative treatment or complication. Data can be from administrative databases, such as claims data, or imputed, using local, regional, or national average costs or charges.
Averted productivity losses	Wages and fringe benefits of participants; average wages of similarly aged persons or of the national average for persons not in the labor force

these costs is that the true economic cost of providing the program should be identified. This is the resource cost of the program, also referred to as the opportunity cost. If this program is undertaken, what other program will we forego? What opportunity must be passed up in order to fund this program? In health, there is often a distinction between *charges* and *costs*. For example, a screening test for diabetes may be billed at $200; however, the cost of providing the test is $150. The $150 figure should be used.

Direct costs include labor costs, often measured by the number of full-time equivalent employees (FTEs) and their wages and fringe benefits. If volunteers will be used, the value of their time should be imputed using either their own wage rates or the average wage rate for similarly skilled work within the community. Other direct costs are supplies and overhead. (Figure 8–4 provides a detailed worksheet for determining direct costs.)

Indirect costs are the other main component of costs. These can be subdivided into five categories. Three of these (time and travel costs, the cost of treating side effects, and the cost of treatment during gained life expectancy) are positive costs and are added to the numerator. The other two (averted treatment costs and averted productivity losses) are negative costs (i.e., benefits) that are subtracted from the numerator because they directly affect the public health budget.

The first category of costs is the time and travel costs to the participants. From a societal standpoint, these costs should be attributed to the program. Often, to obtain these costs, a survey of program participants must be conducted. In addition, if other family members or friends are involved as caregivers to the program participants, their time and travel costs should be included. The second category of indirect costs is the cost of treating side effects. If the intervention causes any side effects, the cost of treating them should be charged to the intervention.

The third component of indirect costs is the cost of treatment during gained life expectancy. If a person's life is extended due to an intervention, he or she will consume additional health care resources in those additional years. Should these costs be added to the numerator of the cost-utility ratio? Proponents of their inclusion argue that these costs are part of the health budget and will affect its future size. Those opposed point out that these persons will also be paying taxes, thus helping to support their additional consumption of health care. Why single out one aspect of their future spending? The U.S. Panel on Cost-Effectiveness did not make a recommendation with respect to this issue,[2] leaving the inclusion of these costs to the discretion of the analyst.

The fourth group of indirect costs is averted treatment costs. These are future treatment costs that will be saved as a result of the intervention. For example, screening for diabetes might identify cases earlier and thus limit or prevent some complications and early mortality. These are complications that will not need to be treated (if prevented) or that will not need to be treated as expensively (if delayed). The incidence of complications with and without the program must be estimated and then multiplied by the costs of treatment to obtain the averted treatment costs.

The fifth category is averted productivity losses. These represent the savings to society from avoiding lost work time. The wages and fringe benefits of participants, of the average wages and fringe benefits of similar persons, or of the average person are used to estimate this negative cost. This cost is used in cost–benefit and cost-effectiveness analyses but not in cost-utility analysis. Benefits in a cost-utility analysis are measured in terms of health utility, which in turn depends upon a person's ability to work and earn an income. Thus, the negative costs of averted productivity losses are included as positive benefits in cost-utility analysis.

Determining benefits.   The next step in the analysis is the identification and measurement of benefits. Here, the selection of the relevant time period is important, especially for public health. The aim of a program or intervention is the improvement of health, so the output to be measured is improved health status. This is a final outcome that may take many years to achieve. Often, a program can only track participants for a brief period of time and any evaluation will, of necessity, measure intermediate outcomes, such as the number of cases identified. In such cases, the literature can often be used to extrapolate the effect of the intermediate outcome on health. For example, suppose that one were evaluating a program designed to increase physical activity levels. Other studies have demonstrated that increased physical activity reduces the risk of cardiac events. These studies can be used to estimate the anticipated final outcomes of the intervention.

The benefits of the program or intervention are the improvement in health and are thus conceptually identical, regardless of the type of economic evaluation. However, the unit of measurement and the specific elements included differs by type of evaluation. Cost–benefit analysis measures the benefits in dollars. Thus, improvements to health must be converted to dollar amounts. If years of life are saved, then these years must be valued in dollars. There are several suggested methods to make this conversion. All of them are subject to heated debate (for an excellent discussion of this topic see Chapter 7 in Drummond, O'Brien, Stoddart, and Torrance[36]).

In response to dissatisfaction with the measurement of health benefits in dollars, particularly the wide range of values found using different methods, some analysts argued for measuring benefits in a naturally occurring health unit, such as years of life saved. This led to the development of cost-effectiveness analysis, which uses a single health measure (years of life saved, cases averted) as the measure of benefits. This has the advantage of not requiring reductions of different outcomes to a single scale, but a single health measure cannot capture all the benefits of most interventions. Most programs yield morbidity and mortality improvements. By being forced to select one health measure, only morbidity or mortality can be used to determine the cost-effectiveness of the project. This underestimates the cost-effectiveness of projects because the total costs are divided by only a portion of the benefits. In addition, only programs with outcomes measured in the same unit (e.g., lives saved) can be compared.

Partly in response to the shortcomings of cost-effectiveness analysis, some analysts argue for the development of a health utility measure of benefits. Such

a measure would combine morbidity and mortality effects into a s
Further, this metric would be based on the utility, or satisfactio.,
status gives to a person. Individuals' self-reports of their valuation of heaɪtɪ
would form the basis of the health utility measure.

Several measures that meet these criteria have been developed. They include
the QALY, the disability-adjusted life year, and the healthy year equivalent. The
most widely used of these is the quality-adjusted life year, or QALY. A QALY
is defined as the amount of time in perfect health that would be valued the same
as a year with a disease or disability. For example, consider a year with end-
stage renal disease, requiring dialysis. Conceptually, the QALY for this condition
is the fraction of a year in perfect health that one would value the same as the
full year with the condition. The QALY assigned to this condition will vary
across persons, with some considering the condition worse than others. If many
individuals are surveyed, however, the average QALY assigned to this condition
can be obtained.

QALYs range from 0 to 1, with 0 defined as dead and 1 as a year in perfect
health. There are several ways to elicit QALY weights from individuals. These
include the visual rating scale, time trade-off method, and the standard gamble.
With the visual rating scale, survey participants are presented with a list of health
conditions. Beside the descriptions of these conditions, there are lines that range
from 0 to 1. Participants are asked to indicate on the lines their QALY valuation
of each health condition by making a mark. A participant might mark "0.6", for
example, for the year with end-stage renal disease.

To measure the benefits in cost-utility analysis, the analyst must identify all
the morbidity and mortality effects of the intervention. These are then weighted
by the appropriate QALY value. QALY values for many diseases and conditions
can be found by searching the literature. Some studies report QALY weights for
only one or a few diseases or conditions (e.g., end-stage renal disease[39]), while
others include tables of QALY values for numerous health states.[40]

For example, suppose that an intervention among 1,000 persons yields fifty
years of life saved. However, these years saved will be lived with some disability.
Review of the literature indicates that this disability has a QALY weight of 0.7.
The benefits of the fifty years of life saved would be valued at 50 · 0.7, or 35
QALYs. Similarly, suppose that the intervention also prevents morbidity among
500 of the participants for one year. If the QALY weight of the averted condition
is 0.9, then (1 − 0.9), or 0.1 QALYs, is saved for each of the 500 persons,
yielding a benefit of 50 QALYs. The total benefits for this program would
be 35 + 50, or 85 QALYs. This summary measure thus combines both the
morbidity and the mortality effects of the intervention. An illustration of the
use of QALYs in measuring the impact of screening for diabetes is shown in
Box 3–2.[41]

Box 3–2. Costs of Screening for Type II Diabetes

Type II diabetes is a chronic disease that usually develops during adulthood and can have multiple complications, including blindness, lower leg amputations, kidney failure, and cardiac problems. These complications can be delayed, minimized, or avoided entirely if the disease is well managed, with good control of blood sugar levels and screening for the onset of complications. Because the disease develops slowly, over a period of years, it is often called the "silent killer": people can live with undetected diabetes for several years, and then the disease is more advanced and the complication rate is higher when they are finally diagnosed. Screening for Type II diabetes is thus an important prevention issue.

In the 1990s the Centers for Disease Control formed the Diabetes Cost-Effectiveness Study Group. As one part of their work the Study Group considered opportunistic screening for Type II diabetes and estimated its cost-effectiveness.[41] The costs and benefits of screening all adults, 25 and over, at a regular physician visit were estimated.

Costs were estimated using national average charges for physician visits, screening tests, and treatments for the various complications. The occurrence of these costs was estimated, using a computer model that followed a hypothetical cohort of 10,000 adults from the age of screening to death. First, the cohort was assumed to have no routine screening. Second, the cohort was assumed to have screening at the next regular physician visit. The two cohorts were then compared with respect to morbidity and morality. Because of the earlier detection and treatment of diabetes in the second cohort, those persons had slightly lower diabetes-related mortality, a lower incidence of complications, and delayed onset of complications.

The benefits of screening come at a cost, though. Screening of the entire adult U.S. population would cost $236,449 per additional year of life saved, or $56,649 per quality-adjusted life year (QALY). These ratios are high relative to other screening programs and other reimbursed interventions. The Task Force also considered subgroups of adults as candidates for screening and found that it is much more cost-effective to screen African-American and younger cohorts. Screening 25 to 34 year olds yields cost-effectiveness ratios of $35,768 per additional life year saved and $13,376 per QALY. For African-Americans aged 25 to 34, the ratios are $2219 per life year and $822 per QALY. Because the American Diabetes Association recommends annual screening of those 45 and older and the economic evaluation was somewhat sensitive to some key assumptions, the Task Force did not definitively recommend changing screening guidelines. However, it did note that the subgroup analyses strongly suggest that younger cohorts, who have a longer life span over which to accrue benefits, and minority cohorts, who have a higher incidence of diabetes, could benefit the most from screening.

Comparing costs to benefits.   Once the costs and benefits of the intervention have been determined, the next step is the construction of the economic evaluation ratio. For a cost-utility analysis, this ratio will be

$$\text{Cost per QALY} = \frac{\text{Direct Costs} + \text{Indirect Costs}}{\text{QALYs}}$$

Using Table 3–2 and substituting the categories of indirect costs into the equation, the numerator can be restated as follows:

$$\text{Costs} = (\text{Direct Costs}) + (\text{Time and Travel Costs})$$
$$+ (\text{Costs of Treating Side Effects}) - (\text{Averted Treatment Costs})$$

Note that the costs of treatment during gained life expectancy have not been included. In addition, averted productivity losses are not subtracted from costs because they enter into the determination of the QALY weights for the condition of interest. The product of a cost-utility analysis, then, is that it costs x for each QALY gained.

In cost–benefit analysis, all the costs and benefits are measured in dollars, so the ratio becomes a single number reflecting the ratio of costs to benefits. For example, a ratio of 1.6 means that it will cost $1.60 for each $1.00 saved. In a cost-effectiveness analysis, benefits are measured in a naturally occurring health unit, so the ratio will be expressed in terms of that unit. For example, a project might cost $25,000 per life saved.

There are two other issues that should be considered in conducting an economic evaluation: discounting and sensitivity analysis. Discounting refers to the conversion of amounts (usually dollars) received over different periods to a common value in the current period. For example, suppose that one were to receive $100 on today's date of each year for five years. Though the amount of money is the same, most people prefer, and value, the nearer payments more than the distant payments. The payment received today will be the most valuable because it can be spent today. One might be willing to trade a slightly smaller payment received today for the payment to be received one year from today, an even slightly smaller payment today for the payment due in two years, etc. Discounting is a formal way to determine the current payments that would be equal in value to distant payments.

In economic evaluation, costs occurring in the future should be discounted to current values. This puts outlays, or expenditures, to be paid in the future on an equal footing with current expenditures. The interest rate should reflect the real rate of growth of the economy, or about 3%. The U.S. Panel on Cost-Effectiveness recommends an interest rate between 0% and 8%,[2] and many studies use rates from 0% to 10%.

Should benefits also be discounted? The U.S. Panel recommends that they should be,[2] arguing that, like money, nearer health states are preferred to farther ones. In other words, saving the life of a person today is more immediate, and hence more valuable, than saving the life of a person thirty years hence.

A final issue to consider is sensitivity analysis. Numerous assumptions are made in constructing the cost-utility ratio. For example, the average effectiveness of an intervention as reported in a review article or meta-analysis may have been used in a cost-utility analysis. The costs and benefits of the intervention depend on its effectiveness and will vary if the effectiveness is higher or lower than anticipated. Sensitivity analysis provides a way to estimate the effect of changing key assumptions used in the economic evaluation.

There are several ways to conduct a sensitivity analysis. All start by identifying the key assumptions and parameters that have been used in the economic evaluation. One method is to construct best-case and worst-case scenarios for the intervention, systematically varying all of the assumptions to favor and then to bias against the intervention. The cost-utility ratio is recalculated for the best-case and worst-case scenarios and then reported along with the original ratio. Another method is to vary the key assumptions one at a time, recalculating the cost-utility ratio each time. A table or figure is usually provided to report the cost-utility ratios for the different assumptions. Yet a third method is to use statistical techniques, specifying the distributions of key parameters and then randomly sampling from those distributions in multiple simulations. This yields a cost-utility ratio with an estimated confidence interval. Regardless of the method used, a sensitivity analysis is a vital component of an economic evaluation. The less variation there is in the cost-utility ratio as key assumptions are varied, the more confident one can be in the results.

Interpreting and using the results. Once the cost-utility (or cost-effectiveness or cost–benefit) ratio has been determined, it must be interpreted. For example, is a program that costs $15,000 per QALY worthwhile? There are two principal ways to interpret and use the cost-utility ratio. The first compares the cost-utility ratio internally to other competing programs; the other uses external references, or places the cost-utility ratio in the context of other economic evaluations.

If several economic evaluations of competing programs have been conducted within an organization, or if information on the cost-utility of several interventions can be obtained, then an internal comparison is warranted. The programs can be ranked from the lowest cost-utility ratio to the highest. Programs with the lowest ratios should generally be funded first, after other considerations are taken into account. For example, a program manager and policy maker also need to consider the amount of resources required to establish and maintain a program, the ethics of various approaches, and the sociopolitical environment.

The alternative way to decide whether a given cost-utility ratio justifies a program is to compare that ratio with other cost-utility ratios. The comparison groups could be either similar or competing programs that have already been funded. Comparison with similar programs helps the practitioner decide whether the proposed program is relatively efficient. If existing screening programs for diabetes cost $25,000 per QALY and the proposed screening program is estimated to cost $15,000 per QALY, then it represents a more efficient screening method.

Comparison with programs that are already funded helps the practitioner argue for funding by insurers or public agencies. For example, the Medicare program provides mammography for women ages 65 and older. This coverage is partially based on economic evaluations of breast cancer screening that estimated cost-utility ratios of between $12,000 and $20,000 per QALY.[42] One could argue, then, that a screening program for diabetes that costs $15,000 per QALY should also be publicly funded. In addition, Garber and Phelps[43] argue that any intervention costing less than $30,000 to $50,000 per QALY is worth funding, based on the average wages of American workers and the context of other publicly funded programs. This threshold value is gaining credence as a justification for interventions.

CHALLENGES AND OPPORTUNITIES IN USING SYSTEMATIC REVIEWS AND ECONOMIC EVALUATIONS

Analytic tools such as systematic reviews and economic evaluation can be extremely valuable for understanding a large body of literature or assessing the cost-effectiveness of an intervention. However, when undertaking or reading a review of the literature or an economic evaluation, several considerations should be kept in mind:

Ensuring Consistency in Quality

Concerns about the quality of systematic reviews have been expressed for over a decade,[11] and there is recent research showing that more than half of epidemiologic reviews are not systematic in reporting methods.[44] Therefore, all systematic reviews require critical appraisal to determine their validity and to establish whether and how they will be useful in practice.[45] Similarly, reviews of the economic evaluation literature have found that studies that are labeled economic evaluations are often only cost studies, only descriptive, or use the methods inappropriately.[46–49]

Addressing Methodological Issues

In both systematic reviews and economic evaluations, there are still areas of debate about the appropriate ways to conduct these evaluations. Analysts can use established methods inappropriately or employ methods still being debated and developed. Three particular areas of concern are as follows: combining studies inappropriately, estimating costs, and measuring benefits.

The first issue, combining studies inappropriately, relates to systematic reviews. Methods of synthesis work well for large effect sizes and randomized designs. When effect sizes are small, with high potential for confounding, it is essential that the component studies are of high quality in both design and execution.

Pertaining to economic evaluation, it is difficult to measure or estimate costs accurately in many public health settings.[50] Sometimes costs are estimated from national or regional data sets, and their local applicability may be questionable. In addition, some programs have high fixed costs, such as equipment or personnel, making it difficult to achieve cost-effectiveness.

Using imperfect metrics for assessing outcomes can present other problems. Some indicators described in this chapter, such as QALYs, are relatively new when it comes to widespread application. Any indicator is imperfect and includes some level of error. When ranking interventions, the QALY score used for a particular condition helps determine the cost-utility ratio. Different QALY values may change an intervention's relative cost-effectiveness. Unfortunately, there are limited studies of QALYs for many conditions and conflicting sets of QALY weights.[51-53]

In addition, measures such as QALYs depend on life expectancy and may discriminate against people who are aged or disabled and have less to gain with an extended lifespan.[54, 55] Another issue regarding QALYs is the question of whose QALYs should be used: a sample of the general population or a sample of the targeted group? This question would be moot if average QALY scores were the same for these two groups, but research indicates that this is rarely the case.[56-58] People with a disease or disability usually gives a higher QALY rating to their condition than does the general public.

Ensuring Effective Implementation

Systematic reviews and economic evaluations can be useful in informing practice and public policy. However, some difficulties can arise in disseminating the results of these types of studies and using the results.

First, there are unclear effects on decision making. In clinical care, there is consistent evidence showing that introduction of new guidelines can have a positive impact on patient care.[59] In population-based public health, there is little published literature on the impacts of systematic reviews on the decision making of policy makers and consumers.[7] Economic evaluations, while used extensively in other countries, particularly those with national health plans, have a checkered history within the United States. For example, the state of Oregon explicitly incorporated economic evaluations into its Medicaid program, but this approach was later abandoned.[60, 61]

A second issue is adapting national or state standards for local needs. Systematic reviews and economic evaluations usually strive to take a national societal perspective. To apply the results of these studies, the practitioner has to consider whether there are specific state or local characteristics that would influence implementation of results from national data. For example, suppose that a policy maker has found a systematic review that supports the use of mass media campaigns to increase physical activity levels. If the city or county in which the policy maker works bans billboard advertising, then the systematic review results would have to be adjusted for this restriction.

Finally, there is the matter of training and accessibility. For many in public health, the key question may be "How does a practitioner learn about or make appropriate use of these tools?" To make better use of systematic reviews, enhanced training is needed both during graduate education and through continuing education of public health professionals working in community settings.

TRANSLATING EVIDENCE INTO RECOMMENDATIONS AND PUBLIC HEALTH ACTION

Several mechanisms and processes have been used recently to translate the findings of evidence-based reviews in clinical and community settings into recommendations for action. Among these are expert panels, practice guidelines, and best practices.

Expert Panels and Consensus Conferences

Systematic reviews and economic evaluations are often developed, refined, and disseminated via expert panels. These panels examine research studies and their relevance to health conditions, diagnostic and therapeutic procedures, planning and health policy, and community interventions.[62-64] Expert panels are conducted by many government agencies, in both executive and legislative branches, as well as by voluntary (i.e., specialty) health organizations such as the American Cancer Society. Ideally, the goal of expert panels is to provide peer review by scientific experts of the quality of the science and scientific interpretations that underlie public health recommendations, regulations, and policy decisions. When conducted well, peer review can provide an important set of checks and balances for the policy-making process.

Consensus conferences are related mechanisms that are commonly used to review scientific evidence. The National Institutes of Health (NIH) have used consensus conferences since 1977 to resolve important and controversial issues in medicine and public health. For example, a highly publicized consensus conference on breast cancer screening was held in the late 1990s to determine whether mammography screening for women ages 40 to 49 years reduces breast cancer mortality.[65] The RAND corporation has examined the application of the NIH consensus methods in nine countries, resulting in suggestions for improving the process.[63]

Four procedural stages of the expert review/consensus development process can be described:[63]

Context. The context for the panel includes the nature of the audience, the topics considered, and how the topics are selected. The issues addressed are limited by the amount of available evidence. In most countries, the topics chosen for consideration by an expert group are selected by a standing committee responsible for assessment of technologies.

Prepanel Process. The prepanel process includes selecting the chairperson, panel members, and presenters. In this stage, background information is prepared. Although oral presentations are important components of a panel meeting, a literature review is common during the prepanel process. The literature review provided to panel members can range from a synthesis of the relevant literature to a comprehensive set of readings on the topic(s) of interest. A common limitation across countries is the lack of a systematic review of the existing literature during the prepanel phase.[63] For some panels, specific questions are circulated in advance of the meeting to frame the scope and direction of the panel. A Delphi process can also be helpful during the prepanel stage (see Chapter 7).[66]

Composition of the Panel. Panels typically range in size from nine to eighteen members. Experts are sought in a variety of scientific disciplines, such as behavioral science, biostatistics, economics, epidemiology, health policy, or medicine, appropriate for the topic(s) under consideration.[62] In all countries studied by RAND, panels were made up of both scientists and lay persons.[63] Panel members should not have financial or professional conflicts of interest.

For many public health issues, it is important to obtain community participation in the expert panel process. The community may be defined geographically, demographically (e.g., women ages 40 years and older), or by disease status (e.g., people who have survived cancer). Community participation may be achieved directly by having one or more community members on the expert panel or in the consensus group. Alternatively, community input may be incorporated by conducting interviews or focus groups and including this information in the packet of materials the panel will consider.

Panel Meeting. This stage involves the activities actually undertaken at the meeting and immediately following it. These details include public and private forums and the group process used to arrive at recommendations and conclusions. Partly because many consensus conferences across countries have been run fairly informally, McGlynn and colleagues suggest that it is important to formalize and document the group process used to make expert decisions.[63] Draft findings from governmental expert panels are often released for public review and comment prior to final recommendations. Resulting statements or recommendations are widely disseminated in an attempt to make an impact on public health practice and research. Expert panels work best when they publish, along with their recommendations, the rationale for their recommendations and the evidence underlying that rationale.

All expert panels are not created equal. Some, such as the U.S. Preventive Services Task Force (USPSTF) and the Task Force on Community Preventive Services, are explicit about linking recommendations to evidence. In general, we would argue that this explicitness is an advantage over more traditional use of "expert opinion" or "global subjective judgment" because "a clear analytic rationale for recommending certain interventions will enhance the ability of . . . users to assess whether recommendations are valid and prudent from their own perspectives . . . make sense in their local contexts . . . and will achieve goals of importance to them."[1] Evidence-based recommendations should therefore be given greater weight.

Practice Guidelines

A guideline is "a formal statement about a defined task or function."[34] In North America, guideline statements are synonymous with recommendations, whereas in parts of Europe, recommendations are stronger than guidelines. In general, practice guidelines offer advice to clinicians, public health practitioners, managed-care organizations, and the public on how to improve the effectiveness and impact of clinical and public health interventions.[67] Guidelines translate the findings of research and demonstration projects into accessible and useable information for public health practice. To influence community and clinical interventions, guidelines are published by many governmental and nongovernmental agencies. For example, guidelines on screening for hypertension have been published periodically by the National High Blood Pressure Education Program since 1972.[68] Using an evidence-based process and consensus, these guidelines provide recommendations to clinicians. Other examples of evidence-based recommendations follow concerning clinical and community preventive services.[64, 69]

Guidelines for Interventions in Clinical Settings.   Over the past decade, several attempts have been made to take a more evidence-based approach to the development of clinical practice guidelines. There are now organizations con-

...outing to the development of evidence-based clinical practice guidelines in prevention in numerous countries, including the United States, Canada, Great Britain, Australia, and in Europe.[70] Two noteworthy efforts are those of the USPSTF and the Canadian Task Force on Preventive Health Care (CTF). The USPSTF and the CTF have collaborated on improving evidence-based clinical prevention for more than sixteen years.[70] For each task force, the primary mandate has been to review and synthesize evidence and to form guidelines focused on primary care clinicians.

The USPSTF is now developing its third edition and represents an excellent example of a process that follows explicit analytic frameworks, takes a systematic approach to data retrieval and extraction, evaluates evidence according to study design and quality, and examines both benefits and harms of intervention.[20] The USPSTF attempts to cast a wide net for each preventive service considered, reviewing multiple types of studies, including randomized controlled trials and observational studies. Recommendations are based in part on a hierarchy of research designs, with the randomized controlled trial receiving the highest score (Table 3–3).[20] When making a recommendation on a particular clinical intervention, the quality of the evidence is placed in a matrix with the net benefit of the intervention. This results in a rating of "A" (strongly recommended); "B" (recommended); "C" (no recommendation); "D" (recommended against); or "I" (insufficient evidence for a recommendation).

Another important resource is the Cochrane Collaboration, an international initiative, begun in 1993 and designed to prepare, maintain, and disseminate systematic reviews of health care interventions.[71] Reviews by the Cochrane Collaboration, updated quarterly, are based exclusively on randomized controlled trials and are available electronically via the Internet or CD-ROM. Cochrane reviews focus primarily on therapeutic interventions, such as the effects of an-

Table 3–3. Hierarchy of Research Designs Used by the U.S. Preventive Services Task Force

Category	Design
I	Evidence obtained from at least one properly randomized controlled trial.
II-1	Evidence obtained from well-designed controlled trials without randomization.
II-2	Evidence obtained from well-designed cohort or case-control analytic studies, preferably from more than one center or research group.
II-3	Evidence obtained from multiple time series with or without the intervention. Dramatic results in uncontrolled experiments (e.g., the results of the introduction of penicillin treatment in the 1940s) could also be regarded as this type of evidence.
III	Opinions of respected authorities, based on clinical experience, descriptive studies and case reports, or reports of expert committees.

Source: from Harris et al.[20]

tidepressants for depression in people with physical illness. The Cochra[ ]tabase catalogs reviews prepared by its members as well as reviews published outside of the collaboration. The database also contains registries on unpublished and ongoing trials that can be used as source data for meta-analyses and other systematic reviews.[4]

Guidelines for Interventions in Community Settings. Recently, an expert panel (the Task Force on Community Preventive Services), supported by the Centers for Disease Control and Prevention, began publishing *The Guide to Community Preventive Services: Systematic Reviews and Evidence-Based Recommendations* (the *Community Guide*).[64] The underlying reasons for developing the *Community Guide* were as follows: (1) practitioners and policy makers value scientific knowledge as a basis for decision making; (2) the scientific literature on a given topic is often vast, uneven in quality, and inaccessible to busy practitioners; and (3) an experienced and objective panel of experts is seldom locally available to public health officials on a wide range of topics.[64] This effort evaluates evidence related to community, or "population-based," interventions and is intended as a complement to the *Guide to Clinical Preventive Services*. It summarizes what is known about the effectiveness and cost-effectiveness of population-based interventions designed to promote health, prevent disease, injury, disability and premature death as well as reduce exposure to environmental hazards.

Sets of related systematic reviews and recommendations are conducted for interventions in broad health topics, organized by behavior (tobacco product use prevention), environment (the sociocultural environment) or specific diseases, injuries, or impairment (vaccine-preventable diseases). A systematic process is followed that includes forming a review development team, developing a conceptual approach focused around an analytic framework, selecting interventions to evaluate, searching for and retrieving evidence, abstracting information on each relevant study, and assessing the quality of the evidence of effectiveness. Information on each intervention is then translated into a recommendation for or against the intervention or a finding of insufficient evidence. For those interventions where there is insufficient evidence of effectiveness, the *Community Guide* provides guidance for further prevention research. In addition, the *Community Guide* takes a systematic approach to economic evaluation, seeking out economic data to complement data on program or policy effectiveness.[46] (The evidence hierarchy for the *Community Guide* is shown in Chapter 2).

To date, evidence reviews and recommendations are available for vaccine-preventable diseases, reducing tobacco use, reducing injury to motor vehicle occupants, diabetes, promoting physical activity, and improving oral health. (Recommendations for promoting tobacco use cessation are shown in Table 3–

Table 3–4. Examples of Recommendations Regarding Interventions to Reduce Exposure to Environmental Tobacco Smoke (ETS) and to Reduce Tobacco Use—Task Force on Community Preventive Services, 2000

Intervention (No. of Qualifying Studies)	Task Force Recommendation Regarding Use	Intervention Description	Key Findings
Strategies to Reduce Exposure to ETS			
Smoking bans and restrictions (n = 10)	Strongly recommended	Bans or limits tobacco smoking in workplaces and public areas (policies, regulations, and laws)	• Effective in reducing workplace exposure to ETS in several different settings and populations • Eight studies documented decreases in daily tobacco consumption among continuing users • Three studies documented increased rates of tobacco-use cessation following implementation of smoking bans
Community education to reduce home ETS exposure (n = 1)	Insufficient evidence	Provides information to persons about reducing ETS exposure in the home	• Insufficient number of studies evaluating the impact of education efforts on reducing ETS exposure in the home environment
Strategies to Reduce Tobacco-Use Initiation			
Increasing the unit price of tobacco products (n = 8)	Strongly recommended	Increases the excise tax on cigarettes (government legislation)	• Effective in reducing both initiation and of tobacco by adolescents • Three studies documented an effect on consumption and use in young adults (18–25 years)
Mass media education to reduce tobacco-use initiation—campaigns (n = 12)	Strongly recommended	Informs viewers through long-term, high-intensity counteradvertising campaigns	• Effective in combination with other interventions such as tobacco product price increases, school-based education, or community education in reducing tobacco use by adolescents • Most qualifying studies measured outcomes in student populations

Source: Centers for Disease Control and Prevention.[72]

Box 3–3. Using Guidelines to Support Health Policy Change for Reducing Alcohol-Related Traffic Fatalities[a]

A systematic review of the evidence of effectiveness of state laws that lower the allowed blood alcohol concentration (BAC) for motor vehicle drivers from 0.1% to 0.08% found that these laws result in reductions of 7% in fatalities associated with alcohol-impaired driving. The review also identified a study that estimated that approximately 500 lives would be saved annually if all states enacted "0.08% BAC laws." Based on this evidence, the Task Force on Community Preventive Services issued a strong recommendation to state policy makers that they consider enacting this type of law.[73]

In response to requests from members of the House Appropriations Committee's Transportation Subcommittee for information about the effectiveness of "0.08% BAC laws," this review and recommendation was summarized by the National Safety Council and provided to the subcommittee in late summer 2000. Based in part on this information, the subcommittee voted to include language in the Transportation Appropriations bill requiring states to enact 0.08% BAC laws or risk losing federal highway construction funds. The House and Senate approved the Transportation Appropriations bill, including the requirement, and the bill was signed into law by President Clinton. Since then, ten states have passed legislation dropping the legal blood alcohol concentration to 0.08% (bringing the total number of states with a 0.08% BAC law to 29).

[a]Contributed by Stephanie Zaza, Centers for Disease Control and Prevention, December 2001.

4.[72]) A full descriptions of the methods and results of each evidence review are found on the *Community Guide* website <http://www.thecommunityguide.org>. Based on dissemination of an early evidence review in the *Community Guide*,[73] health policy has already been positively influenced at the national and state levels (Box 3–3).

"Best Practices" in Public Health

In addition to the analytic approaches discussed thus far, a variety of "best practices" reviews have been conducted and disseminated in recent years. The scope and quality of these reviews vary greatly, making "best practices" an imprecise term. Identification of best practices sometimes occurs when a practitioner informally notes that one intervention activity works better than another.[74] Some researchers have included evidence-based reviews in clinical and community settings under the heading of best practices.[75] Best practices have also involved a grass-roots approach toward injury prevention and traffic safety that engaged local citizens in the decision-making process.[76] Other best practices approaches have been a combination of a strictly evidence-based process and expert opinion on what works. An example here is *Best Practices for Comprehensive Tobacco Control Programs,* developed by the Centers for Disease Control and Prevention.[77] In part, this document was developed in response to demand from states that were deciding how to allocate large sums of litigated damages being paid by the tobacco industry[75] and was largely based on the program successes in states that had established comprehensive and effective tobacco control programs—notably California, Massachusetts, and Oregon.[78–80] Given these variations in how best practices are assembled, readers should carefully scrutinize the process used to develop guidance, particularly when the guidelines do not appear in the peer-reviewed literature.

SUMMARY

This chapter has presented several tools for developing and practicing evidence-based public health, including systematic reviews and economic evaluation. Both are ways to identify, collate, and synthesize what is known about a topic. Systematic reviews give an assessment of state-of-the-art information about a particular intervention and evaluate the efficacy of the intervention. ("Does it work?") Economic evaluation quantifies the costs and benefits of an intervention and provides an assessment of its effectiveness. ("Are the costs reasonable to obtain the likely benefits?") Practice guidelines translate research into information for public health practice. ("What recommendations have been issued by expert panels to address the health condition(s) of interest?")

Each of these techniques is relatively sophisticated and is generally carried out by persons with specialized training (e.g., an economist would conduct a cost-utility analysis). The aim of this chapter has been to explain these techniques to public health practitioners so that they can be educated consumers of these methods.

Key points:

- Systematic reviews and economic evaluations summarize large amounts of information and can provide reliable tools for decision making among public health professionals and policy makers.
- These techniques are relatively sophisticated, but their underlying logic and structure can be understood.
- The outcome of the systematic review process can be a narrative (qualitative) assessment of the literature or a quantitative meta-analysis, and either can be used to inform guideline development.
- Practice guidelines for clinical and community settings are becoming increasingly common and useful.

- Economic evaluation is the comparison of costs and benefits to determine the most efficient allocation of scarce resources.
- Several challenges (inconsistent quality, methodologic issues, difficulties in implementation) should be kept in mind when considering the use of systematic reviews and economic evaluations.

These methods will be increasingly used, especially in times of limited public health resources, and practitioners must be able to understand them so that they can argue for setting appropriate public health priorities.

SUGGESTED READINGS AND WEBSITES

Readings

Drummond MF, O'Brien B, Stoddart GL, Torrance GW. *Methods for the Economic Evaluation of Health Care Programmes*. 2nd ed. New York: Oxford University Press, 1997.

Gold MR, Siegel JE, Russell LB, Weinstein MC. *Cost-Effectiveness in Health and Medicine*. New York: Oxford University Press, 1996.

Haddix AC, Teutsch SM, Shaffer PA, Dunet DO, eds. *Prevention Effectiveness. A Guide to Decision Analysis and Economic Evaluation*. New York: Oxford University Press, 1996.

Mulrow C, Cook D, eds. *Systematic Reviews. Synthesis of Best Evidence for Health Care Decisions*. Philadelphia: American College of Physicians, 1998.

O'Brien B. Principles of economic evaluation for health care programs. *Journal of Rheumatology* 1995;22(7):1399–1402.

Petitti DB. *Meta-analysis, Decision Analysis, and Cost-Effectiveness Analysis: Methods for Quantitative Synthesis in Medicine*. 2nd ed. New York: Oxford University Press, 2000.

Robinson R. Cost-effectiveness analysis. *British Medical Journal*. September 25, 1993; 307(6907):793–795.

Selected Websites

The Cochrane Collaboration <http://www.cochrane.org>. The Cochrane Collaboration is an international organization that aims to help people make well-informed decisions about health care by preparing, maintaining, and promoting the accessibility of systematic reviews of the effects of health care interventions.

Guide to Clinical Preventive Services, Second Edition <http://odphp.osophs.dhhs. gov/pubs/guidecps>. This report is intended for primary care clinicians: physicians, nurses, nurse practitioners, physician assistants, other allied health professionals, and students. It provides recommendations for clinical practice on preventive interventions—screening tests, counseling interventions, immunizations, and chemoprophylactic regimens—for the prevention of more than eighty target conditions. The recommendations in each chapter reflect a standardized review of current scientific evidence and include a summary of published clinical research regarding the clinical effectiveness of each preventive service.

Guide to Community Preventive Services <http://www.thecommunityguide.org>. Under the auspices of the U.S. Public Health Service, a Task Force on Community Preventive Services (the Task Force) is developing a Guide to Community Preventive Services (the Community Guide). The Community Guide will summarize what is known about the effectiveness of population-based interventions for prevention and control. Sections are posted as they become available.

The CUA Database: Standardizing the Methods and Practices of Cost-Effectiveness Analysis, Harvard Center for Risk Analysis, Harvard School of Public Health <http://www.hsph.harvard.edu/organizations/hcra/cuadatabase/intro.html>. This website includes a detailed database of cost-utility analyses. Originally based on the article by Tengs et al. ("Five Hundred Life-Saving Interventions and Their Cost-Effectiveness"),[81] the site is continually updated and expanded.

National Health Service Centre for Reviews and Dissemination <http://www.york.ac.uk/inst/crd>. Maintained by the University of York, this website distributes information and has searchable databases on intervention effectiveness and intervention cost-effectiveness. The NHS Centre for Reviews and Dissemination is devoted to promoting the use of research-based knowledge in health care. Within the website, one can find the NHS Economic Evaluation Database, which provides access to detailed structured abstracts for economic evaluations of healthcare interventions. The database is available free of charge online.

REFERENCES

1. Briss PA, Zaza S, Pappaioanou M, et al. Developing an evidence-based Guide to Community Preventive Services—methods. The Task Force on Community Preventive Services. *American Journal of Preventive Medicine* 2000;18(1 Suppl):35–43.
2. Gold MR, Siegel JE, Russell LB, Weinstein MC. *Cost-Effectiveness in Health and Medicine.* New York: Oxford University Press, 1996.
3. Haddix AC, Teutsch SM, Shaffer PA, Dunet DO, eds. *Prevention Effectiveness. A Guide to Decision Analysis and Economic Evaluation.* 1st ed. New York: Oxford University Press, 1996.
4. Petitti DB. *Meta-analysis, Decision Analysis, and Cost-Effectiveness Analysis: Methods for Quantitative Synthesis in Medicine.* 2nd ed. New York: Oxford University Press, 2000.
5. Zaza S, Wright-De Aguero LK, Briss PA, et al. Data collection instrument and procedure for systematic reviews in the Guide to Community Preventive Services. Task Force on Community Preventive Services. *American Journal of Prevention Medicine* 2000;18(1 Suppl):44–74.
6. Petticrew M. Systematic reviews from astronomy to zoology: Myths and misconceptions. *British Medical Journal* 2001;322(7278):98–101.
7. Bero LA, Jadad AR. How consumers and policy makers can use systematic reviews for decision making. In: Mulrow C and Cook D, (eds.) *Systematic Reviews. Synthesis of Best Evidence for Health Care Decisions.* Philadelphia: American College of Physicians, 1998, pp. 45–54.

8. Cook DJ, Mulrow CD, Haynes B. Synthesis of best evidence for clinical decisions. In: Mulrow C and Cook D, eds. *Systematic Reviews. Synthesis of Best Evidence for Health Care Decisions*. Philadelphia: American College of Physicians, 1998, pp. 5–12.

9. Drummond M, O'Brien B. Economic analysis alongside clinical trials: practical considerations. The Economics Workgroup. *Journal of Rheumatology* 1995;22(7):1418–1419.

10. O'Brien B. Principles of economic evaluation for health care programs. *Journal Rheumatology* 1995;22(7):1399–1402.

11. Mulrow CD. The medical review article: State of the science. *Annals of Internal Medicine* 1987;106(3):485–488.

12. Milne R, Chambers L. Assessing the scientific quality of review articles. *Journal of Epidemiology and Community Health* 1993;47(3):169–170.

13. Woolf SH. Review articles and disclosure of methods. *American Journal of Preventive Medicine* 1991;7(1):53–54.

14. Hutchison BG. Critical appraisal of review articles. *Canadian Family Physician* 1993;39:1097–1102.

15. Oxman AD, Guyatt GH. The science of reviewing research. *Annals of the New York Academy of Science* 1993;703:125–133.

16. Guyatt G, Rennie D, eds. *Users' Guides to the Medical Literature. A Manual for Evidence-Based Clinical Practice*. Chicago: American Medical Association Press, 2002.

17. Mulrow C, Cook D, eds. *Systematic Reviews: Synthesis of Best Evidence for Health Care Decisions*. Philadelphia: American College of Physicians, 1998.

18. Kelsey JL, Petitti DB, King AC. Key methodologic concepts and issues. In: Brownson RC and Petitti DB, (eds.) *Applied Epidemiology: Theory to Practice*. New York: Oxford University Press, 1998, pp. 35–69.

19. Oxman AD, Cook DJ, Guyatt GH. Users' guides to the medical literature. VI. How to use an overview. Evidence-Based Medicine Working Group. *Journal of the American Medical Association* Nov 2, 1994;272(17):1367–1371.

20. Harris RP, Helfand M, Woolf SH, et al. Current methods of the U.S. Preventive Services Task Force. A review of the process. *American Journal of Preventive Medicine* 2001;20(3 Suppl):21–35.

21. Glass GV. Primary, secondary and meta-analysis of research. *Educational Research* 1976;5:3–8.

22. Lau J, Ioannidis JPA, Schmid CH. Quantitative synthesis in systematic reviews. In: Mulrow C and Cook D, (eds.) *Systematic Reviews. Synthesis of Best Evidence for Health Care Decisions*. Philadelphia: American College of Physicians; 1998, pp. 91–101.

23. Wolf FM. *Quantitative Methods for Research Synthesis*. Beverly Hills, CA: Sage Publications, 1986.

24. Ellison R, Zhang Y, McLennan C, Rothman K. Exploring the relation of alcohol consumption to risk of breast cancer. *American Journal of Epidemiology* Oct. 15, 2001;154(8):740–747.

25. Weed DL. Interpreting epidemiological evidence: how meta-analysis and causal inference methods are related. *International Journal of Epidemiology* 2000;29(3):387–390.

26. Greenland S. Can meta-analysis be salvaged? *American Journal of Epidemiology* 1994;140(9):783–787.

27. Cardis E, Gilbert ES, Carpenter L, et al. Effects of low doses and low dose rates of external ionizing radiation: cancer mortality among nuclear industry workers in three countries. *Radiation Research* 1995;142(2):117–132.
28. Lubin JH, Boice JD, Jr., Edling C, et al. Lung cancer in radon-exposed miners and estimation of risk from indoor exposure. *Journal of National Cancer Institute* 1995; 87(11):817–827.
29. Howe GR, McLaughlin J. Breast cancer mortality between 1950 and 1987 after exposure to fractionated moderate-dose-rate ionizing radiation in the Canadian fluoroscopy cohort study and a comparison with breast cancer mortality in the atomic bomb survivors study. *Radiation Research* 1996;145(6):694–707.
30. Samet JM, Burke TA. Epidemiology and risk assessment. In: Brownson RC and Petitti DB, (eds.) *Applied Epidemiology: Theory to Practice.* New York: Oxford University Press, 1998, pp. 137–175.
31. World Health Organization. *Assessment and Management of Environmental Health Hazards.* Vol 89.6. Geneva: WHO/PEP, 1989.
32. Hertz-Picciotto I. Epidemiology and quantitative risk assessment: A bridge from science to policy. *American Journal of Public Health* 1995;85:484–491.
33. U.S. Environmental Protection Agency. Guidelines for carcinogenic risk assessment. *Federal Register* 1986;51:33992–34003.
34. Last JM, ed. *A Dictionary of Epidemiology.* 4th ed. New York: Oxford University Press, 2001.
35. Hatziandreu EI, Koplan JP, Weinstein MC, Caspersen CJ, Warner KE. A cost-effectiveness analysis of exercise as a health promotion activity. *American Journal of Public Health* 1988;78(11):1417–1421.
36. Drummond MF, O'Brien B, Stoddart GL, Torrance GW. *Methods for the Economic Evaluation of Health Care Programmes.* 2nd ed. New York: Oxford University Press, 1997.
37. Weinstein MC, Fineberg HV. *Clinical Decision Analysis.* Philadelphia: WB Saunders Company, 1980.
38. Snider DE, Holtgrave DR, Dunet DO. Decision analysis. In: Haddix AC, Teutsch SM, Shaffer PA and Dunet DO, eds. *Prevention Effectiveness. A Guide to Decision Analysis and Economic Evaluation.* New York: Oxford University Press, 1996, pp. 27–45.
39. Churchill D, Torrance G, Taylor D, et al. Measurement of quality of life in end-stage renal disease: The time trade-off approach. *Clinical and Investigative Medicine* 1987;10(1):14–20.
40. Fryback D, Dasbach E, Klein R, Klein B, Peterson K, Martin P. The Beaver Dam health outcomes study: Initial catalog of health-state quality factors. *Medical Decision Making* 1993;13:89–102.
41. CDC Diabetes Cost-Effectiveness Study Group. The Cost-effectiveness of Screening for Type 2 Diabetes. *JAMA* November 25, 1998;2802(20):1757–1763.
42. Eddy D. *Breast Cancer Screening for Medicare Beneficiaries.* Washington, DC: Office of Technology Assessment, 1987.
43. Garber AM, Phelps CE. Economic foundations of cost-effectiveness analysis. *Journal of Health Economics* February 1997;16(1):1–31.
44. Breslow RA, Ross SA, Weed DL. Quality of reviews in epidemiology. *American Journal of Public Health* 1998;88(3):475–477.

45. Hunt DL, McKibbon KA. Locating and appraising systematic reviews. *Annals of Internal Medicine* 1997;126(7):532–538.
46. Carande-Kulis VG, Maciosek MV, Briss PA, et al. Methods for systematic reviews of economic evaluations for the Guide to Community Preventive Services. Task Force on Community Preventive Services. *American Journal of Preventive Medicine* 2000; 18(1 Suppl):75–91.
47. Zarnke KB, Levine MA, O'Brien BJ. Cost-benefit analyses in the health-care literature: Don't judge a study by its label. *Journal of Clinical Epidemiology* July 1997; 50(7):813–822.
48. Elixhauser A, Luce BR, Taylor WR, Reblando J. Health care CBA/CEA: an update on the growth and composition of the literature. *Medical Care* July 1993;31(7 Suppl): JS1–JS11, JS18–JS149.
49. Udvarhelyi IS, Colditz GA, Rai A, Epstein AM. Cost-effectiveness and cost-benefit analyses in the medicale literature: Are the methods being used correctly? *Annals of Internal Medicine* 1992;116(3):238–244.
50. Petitti DB. Economic evaluation. In: Brownson RC and Petitti DB, (eds.) *Applied Epidemiology: Theory to Practice*. New York: Oxford University Press, 1998, pp. 277–298.
51. Birch S, Gafni A. Cost-effectiveness ratios: In a league of their own. *Health Policy* May 1994;28(2):133–141.
52. Gerard K, Mooney G. QALY league tables: Handle with care. *Health Economics* 1993;2(1):59–64.
53. Drummond M, Torrance G, Mason J. Cost-effectiveness league tables: More harm than good? *Social Science and Medicine* July 1993;37(1):33–40.
54. Harris J. QALYfying the value of life. *Journal of Medical Ethics* 1987;13(3):117–123.
55. Welch HG. Comparing apples and oranges: does cost-effectiveness analysis deal fairly with the old and young? *Gerontologist* 1991;31(3):332–336.
56. Bleichrodt H. Health utility indices and equity considerations. *Journal of Health Economics* February 1997;16(1):65–91.
57. Groot W. Adaptation and scale of reference bias in self-assessments of quality of life. *Journal of Health Economics* 2000;19(3):403–420.
58. Harris RA, Nease RF. The importance of patient preferences for comorbidities in cost-effectiveness analyses. *Journal of Health Economics* February 1997;16(1):113–119.
59. Grimshaw JM, Russell IT. Effect of clinical guidelines on medical practice: a systematic review of rigorous evaluations. *Lancet* 1993;342(8883):1317–1322.
60. Eddy D. Oregon's methods. Did cost-effectiveness analysis fail? *Journal of the American Medical Association* 1991;266(3):417–420.
61. Klevit H, Bates A, Castanares T, Kirk P, Sipes-Metzler P, Wopat R. Prioritization of health care services: a progress report by the Oregon health services commission. *Archives of Internal Medicine* 1991;151:912–916.
62. Brownson RC. Epidemiology and health policy. In: Brownson RC and Petitti DB, (eds.) *Applied Epidemiology: Theory to Practice*. New York: Oxford University Press, 1998, pp. 349–387.
63. McGlynn EA, Kosecoff J, Brook RH. Format and conduct of consensus development conferences. Multination comparison. *International Journal of Technology Assessment in Health Care* 1990;6:450–469.

64. Truman BI, Smith-Akin CK, Hinman AR, et al. Developing the guide to community preventive services—overview and rationale. *American Journal of Preventive Medicine* 2000;18(1S):18–26.
65. Nelson NJ. The mammography consensus jury speaks out. *Journal of the National Cancer Institute* 1997;89(5):344–347.
66. Dalkey N, Helmer O. An experimental application of the Delphi method to the use of experts. *Management Science* 1963;9:458–467.
67. Truman BI, Teutsch SM. Screening in the community. In: Brownson RC and Petitti DB, (eds.) *Applied Epidemiology: Theory to Practice.* New York: Oxford University Press, 1998, pp. 213–247.
68. National Heart Lung and Blood Institute. *The Sixth Report of the Joint National Committee on Prevention, Detection, Evaluation, and Treatment of High Blood Pressure.* Bethesda, MD: National Heart, Lung, and Blood Institute; November 1997. NIH Publication No. 98–4080.
69. Berg AO, Allan JD. Introducing the third U.S. preventive services task force. *American Journal of Preventive Medicine* 2001;20(3 Suppl):3–4.
70. Feightner JW, Lawrence RS. Evidence-based prevention and international collaboration. *American Journal of Preventive Medicine* 2001;20(3 Suppl):5–6.
71. Chalmers I. The Cochrane collaboration: Preparing, maintaining, and disseminating systematic reviews of the effects of health care. *Annals of the New York Academy of Science* Dec. 31, 1993;703:156–163.
72. Centers for Disease Control and Prevention. Strategies for reducing exposure to environmental tobacco smoke, increasing tobacco-use cessation, and reducing initiation in communities and health-care systems. A report on recommendations of the Task Force on Community Preventive Services. *Morbidity and Mortality Weekly Report* November 10, 2000;49(RR-12):1–11.
73. Shults RA, Elder RW, Sleet DA, et al. Reviews of evidence regarding interventions to reduce alcohol-impaired driving. *American Journal of Preventive Medicine* 2001; 21(4 Suppl 1):66–88.
74. Kahan B, Goodstadt M. The interactive domain model of best practices in health promotion: Developing and implementing a best practices approach to health promotion. *Health Promotion Practice* 2001;2(1):43–67.
75. Green LW. From research to "best practices" in other settings and populations. *American Journal of Health Behavior* 2001;25(3):165–178.
76. National Highway Traffic Safety Administration. Safe Communities. A Vision for the Future: A Safe Community in Every Community in America. *NHTSA.* Available at: <http://www.nhtsa.dot.gov/safecommunities/scbestp/>, Accessed November 4, 2001.
77. Centers for Disease Control and Prevention. *Best Practices for Comprehensive Tobacco Control Programs.* Atlanta: Centers for Disease Control and Prevention, National Center for Chronic Disease Prevention and Health Promotion, Office on Smoking and Health, August 1999.
78. California Department of Health Services. *A Model for Change: The California Experience in Tobacco Control.* Sacramento, CA: California Department of Health Services, 1998.
79. Abt Associates. *Independent Evaluation of the Massachusetts Tobacco Control Program: Third Annual Report, January 1994–June 1996.* Cambridge, MA: Abt Associates, 1996.

80. Centers for Disease Control and Prevention. Decline in cigarette consumption following implementation of a comprehensive tobacco prevention and education program—Oregon. *Morbidity and Mortality Weekly Report* 1999;48:140–143.
81. Tengs TO, Adams ME, Pliskin JS, et al. Five-hundred life-saving interventions and their cost-effectiveness. *Risk Analysis* 1995;15(3):369–390.

4

Developing an Initial Statement of the Issue

> The uncreative mind can spot wrong answers. It takes a creative mind to spot wrong questions.
>
> —A. Jay

The first step in an evidence-based process is to develop a concise statement of the issue being considered. A clear articulation of the problem at hand will enhance the likelihood that a systematic and focused planning process can be followed, leading to successful outcomes. A clear statement of the issue provides a concrete basis for a priority setting process that is objective and then for program planning, intervention, and evaluation.[1] A fully articulated issue statement includes a complete description of the problem, potential solutions, data sources, and health-related outcomes. While this may seem straightforward, developing a sound issue statement can be challenging. In fact, the development of well-stated and answerable clinical questions has been described as the most difficult step in the practice of evidence-based medicine.[2]

Issue statements can be initiated in at least three different ways. They might be part of a section on background and objectives of a grant application for external support of a particular intervention or program. Since this is generally the first portion of a grant application to be viewed by funders, a clear delineation of the issue under consideration is crucial. An issue statement might also be in response to a request from an administrator or an elected official about a particular issue. For example, a governor might and seek input from agency personnel on a specific problem. Your task might be to develop a politically and scientifically acceptable issue statement within a short time period in response. Or, a program or agency might define issues as a result of a needs assessment or as part of a strategic planning process that could take several months to implement and evaluate. Each scenario demonstrates a different set of reasons and circumstances for defining a particular public health issue. In all cases, it is essential that the initial statement of the issue be clear, articulate, and well-understood by all members of the public health team, as well as other relevant parties.

This chapter is divided into two major sections. The first examines some lessons and approaches that can be learned from the processes of needs assessment and strategic planning. The second describes a systematic approach to developing an issue statement by breaking it into four component parts: background/epidemiologic data; questions about the program or policy; solutions being considered; and potential outcomes. It should be remembered that an initial issue statement is likely to evolve as more information is gathered in the course of program implementation and policy development.

BACKGROUND

Developing a concise and useful issue statement can be informed by the processes of needs assessment and strategic planning. In a needs assessment, issues emerge and are defined in the process of determining the health needs or desires of a population. In strategic planning, the identification of key strategic issues helps define the priorities and direction for a group or organization. In addition, issue definition is closely linked with the objective setting steps involved in developing an action plan for a program (Chapter 8) and also forms part of the foundation of an effective evaluation strategy (Chapter 9).

Key Aspects of Needs Assessment

Needs assessments will be discussed in more detail in the context of evaluation in Chapter 9. In brief, a needs assessment is "a systematic set of procedures undertaken for the purpose of setting priorities and making decisions about program or organizational improvement and allocation of resources. The priorities are based on identified needs."[3] A needs assessment may involve a variety of different data types, including epidemiologic (quantitative) data, qualitative information, data on health inequalities, and patterns of health resource utilization.[4]

The initial aspects of a needs assessment are especially pertinent when defining an issue or problem. A typical needs assessment would begin by considering sources of baseline or background data on a health problem or a community. These sources might include primary and/or secondary data. Primary data involves collection of new information for a particular program or study through such methods as a community survey, interviews, focus groups, etc. Collection of primary data often occurs over a relatively long period of time, sometimes years, although a local community assessment survey can be done in three to six months. Needs assessments often rely on secondary data sources—that is, data routinely collected at a local, state or national level. The biggest advantages of using secondary data rather than collecting primary data are time and cost.[5] Many government, university, and nonprofit agencies spend years and many dollars in collecting and maintaining data. These agencies also add technical expertise to data collection that helps ensure that data are high quality. Several important sources of secondary data are readily available and are listed with their websites at the end of this chapter. One disadvantage of secondary data is that detailed local information may not be available for smaller or less populous areas. Community health assessments often use a mix of primary and secondary data. In addition to quantitative secondary data on morbidity, mortality, and health behaviors, they may make use of qualitative primary data collected via interviews or focus group methods.[6]

Key Aspects of Strategic Planning

Strategic planning is a disciplined effort to produce decisions and actions that shape and guide what an organization is, what it does, and why it does it.[7] It is a continuous process for identifying intended future outcomes and how success will be measured, often with a three- to five-year time horizon. A complete discussion of strategic planning benefits and methods is available elsewhere.[7-10] Rational strategic planning is based on three deceptively simple questions: "Where are we?"; "Where do we want to be?"; and "How do we get there?"[10] In this section, specific aspects that help shape issue definition within an evidence-based public health framework are reviewed.

In many senses, problem definition is similar to the early steps in a strategic planning process, which often involve reaching consensus on the mission and values of the organization, analyzing the internal and external environments, involving people affected by the plan in the process, and creating a common vision for the future. As noted in Chapter 1, the public health environment is ever-changing and shaped by new science and information, policies, and social forces. In particular, the early phases of a strategic planning process often involve an environmental assessment. This assessment may include an analysis of political, economic, social and technological (PEST) trends in the larger environment. Such an analysis is important in order to understand the context in which specific problems are embedded and within which they must be addressed. A SWOT analysis (identification of an organization's internal strengths and weaknesses and external opportunities and threats) is often prepared as well (Figure 4–1). The SWOT analysis brings the resources and gaps (strengths and

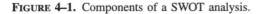

Positive   Negative

Internal	Strengths	Weaknesses
External	Opportunities	Threats

Figure 4–1. Components of a SWOT analysis.

weaknesses) within the organization into focus and assesses the impact of external forces (opportunities and threats). As an issue becomes more clearly defined using the methods detailed in the next section, it is important to remember the context in which the issue is being addressed. Some of the questions and areas that may be considered early in an environmental assessment are shown in Table 4–1.[11] Later, when strategies are known, a comprehensive assessment of resources—financial and nonfinancial—is needed. A well-done needs assessment and/or environmental analysis can increase the likelihood of asking the right questions that will later guide an evidence-based process.

Table 4–1. Important Questions to Consider in an Environmental Analysis

Area of Interest	Questions to Consider
Internal assessment	Is this issue relevant to the mission and values of the organization? What, if anything, are we already doing to address the issue? Does the organization have the desire and ability to address this issue? Who in the agency has an interest in seeing the issue addressed? If so, how high is the priority of this issue for the organization?
External assessment	Will the community accept and support addressing this issue? Are there government regulations and other legal factors affecting the issue? Have the views of each important stakeholder been taken into account? Are there other external groups addressing this issue with success or lack of success (both current and in the past)?

Source: adapted from Timmreck.[11]

DIVIDING AN ISSUE INTO ITS COMPONENT PARTS

When beginning to define an issue, several fundamental questions should be asked and answered:

- What was the basis for the initial statement of the issue? This may include the social/political/health circumstances at the time the issue was originated, and how it was framed. This provides the context for the issue.
- Who was the originator of the concern? The issue may have developed internally within an organization or may be set as an issue by a policy maker or funder.
- Should/could the issue be stated in the epidemiologic context of person (How many people are affected and who are they?), place (What is the geographic distribution of the issue?), and time (How long has this issue been a problem? What are anticipated changes over time?)?[12]
- Is there a consensus among stakeholders that the problem is properly stated?

This section will begin to address these and other questions that one may encounter an initial issue statement is developed. A sound issue statement may draw on multiple disciplines, including biostatistics, epidemiology, health communication, health education, planning, and policy analysis. An issue statement should be stated as a quantifiable question (or series of questions), leading to an analysis of root causes or likely intervention approaches. It should also be unbiased in its anticipated course of action. Figure 4–2 describes the progression

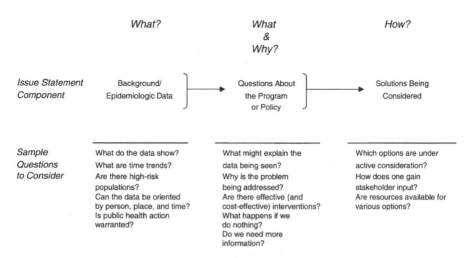

FIGURE 4–2. A sequential framework for understanding the key steps in developing an issue statement.

of an issue statement along with some of the questions that are crucial to answer. One question along the way is "Do we need more information?" The answer to that question is nearly always yes, so the challenge becomes where to find the most essential information efficiently. It is also essential to remember that the initial issue statement is often the "tip of the iceberg" and that getting to the actual causes of and solutions to the problem takes considerable time and effort. Causal frameworks (aka, analytic framework; see Chapter 7) are often useful in mapping out an issue.

Issue Components

The four key components of an issue statement include

1. Background/epidemiologic data
2. Questions about the program or policy
3. Solutions being considered
4. Potential outcomes

Initially, each of these four components should be framed succinctly, in a maximum of one paragraph each. As intervention approaches are later decided upon, these brief initial statements will be refined and expanded into more complete protocols.

An example of the four components of an issue statement, along with potential data sources, is presented in Table 4–2. The section on *background and epidemiologic data* generally presents what is known of the descriptive epidemiology of a public health issue. This includes data on person, place, and time that are often presented as rates or percentage changes over time. It is often useful to present a visual display of the epidemiologic data. For example, Figure 4–3 shows that recent U.S. trends in mammography screening differ substantially for lower-income compared with higher-income women.[13] It is often useful to examine ethnic variations in a preventable risk factor over some time period (Figure 4–4). If available, qualitative information may also be presented with the background statement. For example, focus group data may be available that demonstrates a particular attitude or belief toward a public health issue. The concepts presented earlier in this chapter related to needs assessment are often useful in assembling background data. In all cases, it is important to specify the source of the data so that the presentation of the problem is credible.

In considering the *questions about the program or policy*, the search for effective intervention options (our "Type II evidence") begins. You may want to undertake a strategic planning process in order to generate a set of potentially

Table 4-2. Examples of an Initial Issue Statement for Breast Cancer Control

Component	Example Statement/Questions	Potential Data Sources
Background/epidemiologic data	Based on data from the BRFSS, only 45% of California women aged 50 years and older are receiving mammography screening each year. Rates of screening have remained constant over the past five years and are lowest among lower income women.	CDC WONDER CDC BRFSS data State vital statistics State and local surveillance reports
Questions about the program or policy	Do we understand why screening rates are lower among lower-income women? Why is this a problem? Are there examples in the scientific literature of effective programs to increase the rate of mammography screening among women? Are there similar programs targeted to lower income women? Are there cost-effectiveness studies of these interventions? Have health policies been enacted and evaluated that have had a positive impact on mammography screening rates?	MEDLINE/PubMed Professional meetings Guidelines Legislative records
Solutions being considered	Numerous solutions have been proposed, including: (1) increased funding for mammography screening among low income women; (2) a mass media campaign to promote screening; (3) education of health care providers on how to effectively counsel women for mammography screening; and (4) a peer support program that involves the target audience in the delivery of the intervention	Program staff Policymakers Advisory groups Women with breast cancer
Potential outcomes	Rate of breast cancer mortality Rate of breast cancer mortality among low income women Rate of mammography screening Rate of counseling for mammography among primary care providers	CDC WONDER CDC BRFSS data HEDIS data Program records

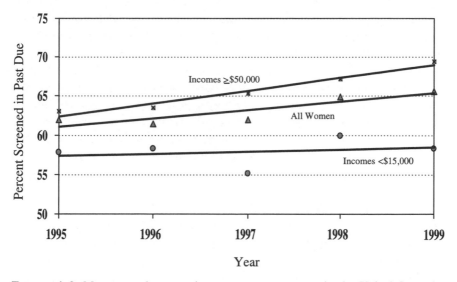

FIGURE 4–3. Mammography screening rates among women in the United States by income group, 1995–1999.[13]

effective program options that could address the issue. The term *program* is defined broadly to encompass any organized public health action, including direct service interventions, community mobilization efforts, policy development and implementation, outbreak investigations, health communication campaigns, health promotion programs, and applied research initiatives.[12] The programmatic issue being considered may be best presented as a series of questions that a public health team will attempt to answer. It may be stated in the context of an intervention program, a health policy, cost-effectiveness, or managerial challenge. For an intervention, you might ask, "Are there effective intervention programs in the literature to address risk factor X among population Y?" A policy question would consider "Can you document the positive effects of a health policy that was enacted and enforced in State X?" In the area of cost-effectiveness, it might be "What is the cost of intervention Z per year of life saved?" And a managerial question would ask, "What are the resources needed to allow us to effectively initiate a program to address issue X?"

As the issue statement develops, it is often useful to consider *potential solutions*. However, several caveats are warranted at this early phase. First, solutions generated at this phase may or may not be evidence-based, since all the information may not be in hand. Also, the program ultimately implemented is likely to differ from the potential solutions discussed at this stage. Finally, solutions noted in one population or region may or may not be generalizable to other populations. There is a natural tendency to jump too quickly to solutions before the background and programmatic focus of a particular issue is well defined. In Table 4–3, potential solutions are presented that are largely developed from the efforts of the *Guide to Community Preventive Services*, an evidence-based guideline described in Chapter 3.[14–16]

When framing *potential solutions* of an issue statement, it is useful to consider whether a "high-risk" or population strategy is warranted. The high-risk strategy focuses on individuals who are most at risk for a particular disease or risk factor.[17,18] Focusing an early detection program on lower-income individuals who have the least access to screening, for example, is a high-risk approach. A population strategy is employed when the risk being considered is widely diffused across a population. A population strategy might involve conducting a mass media campaign to increase early detection among all persons at risk. In practice, these two approaches are not mutually exclusive. The health goals for the United States, for example, call for elimination of health disparities (a high-risk approach) and also target overall improvements in important risk factors such as cigarette smoking, physical inactivity, and unhealthy eating (a population approach).[19] Data and available resources can help in determining whether a population approach, a high-risk strategy, or both is warranted.

Although it may seem premature to consider *potential outcomes* before an intervention approach is decided upon, an initial scan of outcomes is often valuable at this stage. It is especially important to consider the answer to the questions, "What outcome do we want to achieve in addressing this issue? What would a good or acceptable outcome look like?" This process allows you to consider potential short- and longer-term outcomes. It also helps shape the choice of possible solutions and determines the level of resources that will be required to address the issue. For many U.S. public health issues (e.g., numerous environmental health exposures), data do not readily exist for needs assessment and evaluation at a state or local level. Long-term outcomes (e.g., mortality rates) that are often available are not useful for planning and implementing programs with a time horizon of a few years. A significant challenge to be discussed in later chapters is the need to identify valid and reliable intermediate outcomes for public health programs.

Importance of Stakeholder Input

As the issue definition stage continues, it is often critical to obtain the input of "stakeholders." Stakeholders, or key players, are individuals or agencies with a vested interest in the issue at hand.[5] When addressing a particular health policy, policy makers are especially important stakeholders.[20] Stakeholders can also be individuals who would potentially receive, use, and benefit from the program or policy being considered. In particular, three groups of stakeholders are relevant:[12]

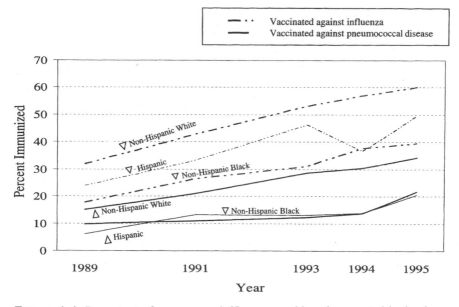

FIGURE 4–4. Percentage of persons aged 65 years or older who reported having been vaccinated against influenza, by race and Hispanic origin, 1989–1995.

Note: Hispanics may be of any race. For influenza, the percent vaccinated consists of persons who reported having a flu shot during the past 12 months. For pneumococcal disease, the percent refers to persons who reported ever having a pneumonia vaccination.

Reference population: These data refer to the civilian noninstitutional population.

Source: National Health Interview Survey.

1. Those involved in program operations, such as sponsors, coalition partners, administrators, and staff;
2. Those served or affected by the program, including clients, family members, neighborhood organizations, and elected officials;
3. Primary users of the evaluation—people who are in a position to do or decide something regarding the program. (These individuals may overlap with the first two categories.)

Table 4–4 shows how the considerations and motivations of various stakeholders can vary.[21] These differences are important to take into account while garnering stakeholder input.

An example of the need for stakeholder input can be seen in Box 4–1. In this case, there are likely to be individuals and advocacy groups with strong feelings regarding how best to reduce infant mortality. Some of the approaches, such as increasing funding for family planning, may be controversial. As described in

Table 4-3. Example of an Initial Issue Statement for Influenza Vaccination among People Aged 65 Years and Older

Component	Example Statement/Questions	Potential Data Sources
Background/epidemiologic data	Based on the National Health Interview Survey, rates of influenza immunization among people aged 65 years and older have doubled over the past six years (Figure 4–4). Despite this increase, rates are below those recommended and are particularly low among certain racial and ethnic minority groups.	National Health Interview Survey US Administration on Aging State vital statistics State and local surveillance reports
Questions about the program or policy	How effective are vaccinations in reducing hospitalizations and deaths due to influenza? What are historical rates of influenza vaccination among people aged 65 years and older? Are all income and racial/ethnic groups affected equally? Are there public health interventions that have been documented to increase coverage of influenza vaccination among people aged 65 years and older?	MEDLINE Healthy People 2010, state health plans Professional meetings Guidelines Legislative records
Solutions being considered	Numerous solutions have been proposed, including: (1) educational programs for the target population; (2) client reminder/recall interventions delivered via telephone or letter; (3) home visits for socioeconomically disadvantaged populations; (4) community mass media programs; and (5) programs to expand vaccination access in health care settings.	Program staff Guidelines Policymakers Advisory groups (e.g., AARP)
Potential outcomes	Rates of immunization Rates of influenza incidence (a reportable disease) Rates of influenza vaccination among various Health Maintenance Organizations Rates of mortality due to influenza	CDC WONDER CDC BRFSS data HEDIS data Program records

Table 4–4. Major Health Policy Considerations among Stakeholders
in the United States

Stakeholder	Consideration
Politicians	The cost of medical care is too high.
	There are too many uninsured Americans.
	The Medicare program is going bankrupt.
	Doctors charge too much.
	There are too many doctors (A rural politician might say the opposite.).
Health-care professionals	There is an overutilization of health services, especially in certain areas of the country; and an underutilization of some services in other areas.
	There is an increase in the "intensity" of health services. i.e., technology that results in increased costs.
	The effect of improved health services over time has been decreased death rates and increased life expectancy.
	More efficient health care delivery will reduce health care costs.
Public health advocates	The health of the American public has improved substantially as demonstrated by declining death rates and longer life expectancy.
	Major public health programs have been successful in reducing key risk factors such as cigarette smoking, control of hypertension, and dietary changes.
	Accessibility and distribution of health services have improved over time.
	There are millions of Americans who lack heath care coverage.
	Environmental monitoring and control have helped decrease morbidity and mortality.
	Prevention is the cornerstone of effective health policy.
Consumers	Personal and out-of-pocket health care costs are too high.
	Quality medical care is often not provided.
	There are substantial risks to the public from "involuntary" environmental hazards such as radiation, chemicals, food additives, and occupational exposures.
	The medical establishment suppresses new therapies.

Source: Adapted from Kuller.[21]

other parts of this book, there are several different mechanisms for gaining
stakeholder input, including:

- Interviews of leaders of various voluntary and nonprofit agencies that have an interest in this issue
- Focus groups with clients who may be served by various interventions
- Newspaper content analysis of clippings that describe previous efforts to enhance health

---

Box 4–1. Reducing Infant Mortality in Texas

For the newly hired director of maternal and child health at the Texas Department of Health, the issue of disparities in infant mortality rates is of high interest. You have been charged by the governor with developing a plan for reducing the rate of infant mortality. This plan must be developed within six months and implemented within a year.

The data show that rates of infant mortality in Texas have been relatively stable over the past five years. The rate among whites is currently 6.4 per 1,000 live births and the rate among African Americans is 11.6 per 1,000 live births, a relative difference of 81%.

Program staff, policy makers, and advisory groups (stakeholders) have proposed numerous intervention options, including: (1) increased funding for family planning services; (2) a mass media campaign to encourage women to seek early prenatal care; and (3) global policies that are aimed at increasing health care access for pregnant women. Program personnel face a significant challenge in trying to obtain adequate stakeholder input within the time frame set out by the governor. You have to decide on the method(s) for obtaining adequate and representative feedback from stakeholders in a short time frame.

Some of the issues you need to consider include the following:

- The role of the government and the role of the private sector in reducing infant mortality
- The positions of various religious groups on family planning
- The key barriers facing women of various ethnic backgrounds when obtaining adequate prenatal care and
- The views of key policy makers in Texas who will decide the amount of public resources available for your program

---

SUMMARY

This chapter is a transition point to numerous other chapters in this book. It begins a sequential and systematic process for evidence-based decision making in public health. The extent to which a practitioner may undergo a full-fledged baseline needs assessment is often dependent on time and resources. It should also be remembered that public health is a team sport, and review and refinement of an initial issue statement with one's team is essential. Several other key points from this chapter:

- There are multiple reasons to draft an issue statement early in an evidence-based process.
- An environmental assessment will help in understanding the context for a program or policy.
- Breaking an issue into its component parts (background/epidemiologic data,

questions about the program or policy, solutions being considered, and potential outcomes) will enhance the process.

- Stakeholder input is essential for informing the approaches to solving many public health problems.

SUGGESTED READINGS AND WEBSITES

Readings

Bryson JM. *Strategic Planning for Public and Nonprofit Organizations. A Guide to Strengthening and Sustaining Organizational Achievement*. San Francisco: Jossey-Bass Publishers, 1995.

Ginter PM, Swayne LM, Duncan WJ. *Strategic Management of Health Care Organizations*. 3rd ed. Malden, MA: Blackwell Publishers Inc., 1998.

Rose G. *The Strategy of Preventive Medicine*. Oxford, UK: Oxford University Press, 1992.

Timmreck TC. *Planning, Program Development, and Evaluation. A Handbook for Health Promotion, Aging and Health Services*. Boston: Jones and Bartlett Publishers, 1995.

Selected Websites

CDC BRFSS <http://www.cdc.gov/nccdphp/brfss> The BRFSS is an ongoing data collection program that is conducted in all states, the District of Columbia, and three U.S. territories. The BRFSS, the world's largest telephone survey, tracks health risks in the United States. Information from the survey is used to improve the health of the American people. CDC has developed a standard core questionnaire for states to use to provide data that could be compared across states.

CDC WONDER <http://wonder.cdc.gov> CDC WONDER is an easy-to-use system that provides a single point of access to a wide variety of CDC reports, guidelines, and numeric public health data. It can be valuable in public health research, decision making, priority setting, program evaluation, and resource allocation.

The Community Health Status Indicators (CHSI) Project <http://www.communityhealth.hrsa.gov> The CHSI Project was launched in response to grassroots requests from local health officials for health data at the local level. The CHSI project team created 3,082 reports of health status indicators, one for each county in the nation. Secondary data were used to create these reports.

Partners in Information Access for Public Health Professionals <http://www.nnlm.nlm.nih.gov/partners> A collaborative project to provide public health professionals with timely, convenient access to information resources to help them improve the health of the American public.

REFERENCES

1. Vilnius D, Dandoy S. A priority rating system for public health programs. *Public Health Reports* 1990;105(5):463–470.

2. Sackett DL, Straus SE, Richardson WS, Rosenberg W, Haynes RB. *Evidence-Based Medicine. How to Practice and Teach EBM.* 2nd ed. Edinburgh: Churchill Livingston, 2000.

3. Witkin BR, Altschuld JW. *Conducting and Planning Needs Assessments. A Practical Guide.* Thousand Oaks, CA: Sage Publications; 1995, p. 4.

4. Wright J, Williams R, Wilkinson JR. Development and importance of health needs assessment. *British Medical Journal* 1998;316(7140):1310–1313.

5. Soriano FI. *Conducting Needs Assessments. A Multidisciplinary Approach.* Thousand Oaks, CA: Sage Publications, 1995.

6. Gilmore GD, Campbell MD. *Needs Assessment Strategies for Health Education and Health Promotion.* 2nd ed. Madison, WI: Browns & Benchmark Publishers, 1996.

7. Bryson JM. *Strategic Planning for Public and Nonprofit Organizations. A Guide to Strengthening and Sustaining Organizational Achievement.* San Francisco: Jossey-Bass Publishers; 1995.

8. Ginter PM, Swayne LM, Duncan WJ. *Strategic Management of Health Care Organizations.* 3rd ed. Malden, MA: Blackwell Publishers Inc., 1998.

9. Ginter PM, Duncan WJ, Capper SA. Keeping strategic thinking in strategic planning: Macro-environmental analysis in a state health department of public health. *Public Health* 1992;106:253–269.

10. Hadridge P. Strategic approaches to planning health care. In: Pencheon D, Guest C, Melzer D, and Muir Gray JA, eds. *Oxford Handbook of Public Health Practice.* Oxford: Oxford University Press; 2001, pp. 342–347.

11. Timmreck TC. *Planning, Program Development, and Evaluation. A Handbook for Health Promotion, Aging and Health Services.* Boston: Jones and Bartlett Publishers, 1995.

12. Centers for Disease Control and Prevention. Framework for program evaluation in public health. *Morbidity and Mortality Weekly Report* 1999;48(RR–11):1–40.

13. Centers for Disease Control and Prevention. Behavioral Risk Factor Surveillance System website. <http://www.cdc.gov/nccdphp/brfss/> 2001.

14. Briss PA, Rodewald LE, Hinman AR, et al. Reviews of evidence regarding interventions to improve vaccination coverage in children, adolescents, and adults. The Task Force on Community Preventive Services. *American Journal of Preventive Medicine* 2000;18(1 Suppl):97–140.

15. Task Force on Community Preventive Services. Vaccine preventable diseases: improving vaccination coverage in children, adolescents, and adults. *Morbidity and Mortality Weekly Report* 1999;48(RR-8):1–16.

16. Truman BI, Smith-Akin CK, Hinman AR, et al. Developing the guide to community preventive services—overview and rationale. *American Journal of Preventive Medicine* 2000;18(1S):18–26.

17. Rose G. Sick individuals and sick populations. *International Journal of Epidemiology* 1985;14(1):32–38.

18. Rose G. *The Strategy of Preventive Medicine.* Oxford: Oxford University Press, 1992.

19. U.S. Dept. of Health and Human Services. *Healthy People 2010. Vol. II. Conference Edition.* Washington, DC: U.S. Dept. of Health and Human Services, 2000.

20. Sederburg WA. Perspectives of the legislator: allocating resources. *Morbidity and Mortality Weekly Report* 1992;41(Suppl):37–48.

21. Kuller LH. Epidemiology and health policy. *American Journal of Epidemiology* 1988;127(1):2–16.

5

Quantifying the Issue

The new source of power is not money in the hands of a few but information in the hands of many.

—John Naisbitt

As discussed in Chapter 4, the needs assessment must include the health condition or risk factor being considered, the population affected, the size and scope of the problem, prevention opportunities, and potential stakeholders. This task requires basic epidemiologic skills to obtain additional information about the frequency of the health condition or risk factor in an affected population. For example, if there is concern about excess disease (a term that will be used as a generic synonym for any health condition or risk factor in this chapter) in a population, we must determine the parameters that define the population at risk. Should we focus on the total population, or restrict the population to males or females of certain ages? Once the population is defined, we must estimate the frequency of disease present in the population. Can we determine the number of diseased persons from existing public health surveillance systems, or must we conduct a special survey of the defined population? Once disease rates are computed, do we see any patterns of disease that identify or confirm subgroups within the defined population that have the highest disease rates? Finally, can we use this information to develop and evaluate the effectiveness of new public health programs?

This chapter provides an overview of the principles of epidemiology that relate to public health practice. It focuses primarily on methods used to measure and characterize disease frequency in defined populations. It includes information about public health surveillance systems and currently available data sources via the Internet. It also provides an overview of the methods used to evaluate the effectiveness of new public health programs that are designed to reduce the prevalence of risk factors and the disease burden in target populations.

BASIC OVERVIEW OF DESCRIPTIVE EPIDEMIOLOGY

Epidemiology is commonly defined as the study of the distribution and determinants of disease or injury in human populations. In a more comprehensive definition relevant to public health practice, Terris[1] stated that epidemiology is the study of the health of human populations for the following purposes:

1. To discover the agent, host, and environmental factors that affect health, in order to provide a scientific basis for the prevention of disease and injury and the promotion of health
2. To determine the relative importance of causes of illness, disability, and death, in order to establish priorities for research and action
3. To identify those sections of the population that have the greater risk from specific causes of ill health, in order to direct the indicated action appropriately
4. To evaluate the effectiveness of health programs and services in improving the health of the population

The first two functions provide etiologic (or Type I) evidence to support causal associations between modifiable and nonmodifiable risk factors and specific diseases, as well as the relative importance of these risk factors when establishing priorities for public health interventions. The third function focuses on the frequency of disease in a defined population and the subgroups within the population to be targeted with public health programs. The last function provides experimental (or Type II) evidence that supports the relative effectiveness of specific public health interventions to address a particular disease.

The terms *descriptive epidemiology* and *analytic epidemiology* are commonly used when presenting the principles of epidemiology. Descriptive epidemiology encompasses methods for measuring the frequency of disease in defined populations. These methods can be used to compare the frequency of disease within and between populations in order to identify subgroups with the highest frequency of disease and to observe any changes that have occurred over time. Analytic epidemiology focuses on identifying essential factors that influence the prevention, occurrence, control, and outcome of disease. Methods used in analytic epidemiology are necessary for identifying new risk factors for specific diseases and for evaluating the effectiveness of new public health programs designed to reduce the disease risk for target populations.

Estimating Disease Frequency

Although one way to measure disease frequency is to count the number of diseased persons, a better method is to estimate the rate of disease in a defined population over time. The rate is computed by dividing the number of persons with the disease of interest by the number of persons at risk of developing the disease during a specified period. For example, 3,902 women residing in Missouri were diagnosed with breast cancer during 1998. Thus, the breast cancer rate equals 3,902 cases of breast cancer divided by 2,805,259 women residing in Missouri on July 1, 1998 (or the midpoint of the year). The rate is 0.00139 breast cancers per woman, or 139 breast cancers per 100,000 women per year. Here, we use data from the Missouri Cancer Registry to identify all pathology-confirmed breast cancers that occurred among women who were residing in Missouri during 1998 and data from the United States Census Bureau to estimate the number of women of all ages residing in Missouri on July 1, 1998.)

Although a disease rate represents the number of cases of disease that occurs in the population during a specified period, it is very difficult to follow each person in the population for the same amount of time over long periods. A more precise way of dealing with persons who move in or out of the population during the study period is to estimate "person-time" for the population at risk, or the amount of time that each person in the population is free from disease during the study period. In our example, every woman residing in Missouri from January 1 to December 31, 1998, contributes one person-year if she is not diagnosed with breast cancer during the study period. Each woman diagnosed with breast cancer during the study period, or whose breast cancer status is unknown, contributes a fraction of a person-year, based on the amount of time that elapsed from January 1, 1998, to her date of diagnosis or departure from the study population, respectively. The sum of every woman's person-time contribution equals the total number of person-years for this population during the one-year study period. If we are unable to determine the amount of person-time for each woman in the study population, the total person-years (2,805,259 person-years) can be estimated by multiplying the estimated number of women in the state at the midpoint of the year (2,805,259) times the duration of the study period (1 year).

Disease rates should measure the occurrence of disease in the population at risk. In other words, the rate should reflect the incidence (the number of new cases of disease among members of the population who are at risk of developing the disease) and not the prevalence (the number of existing cases of disease among surviving members of the population) of disease in the population. Both measures of disease frequency are useful. Prevalence provides essential information when planning health services for the total number of persons who are living with the disease in the community, whereas incidence reflects the true rate of disease occurrence in the same population.

Although incidence rates are ideal for measuring the occurrence of disease in a population for a specified period, they are often not available. In this case, it may be prudent to use cause-specific mortality rates based on the number of deaths from the disease of interest that occurs in the population during the same study period. Mortality rates are often used in lieu of incidence rates, but are only reasonable surrogate measures when the disease is highly fatal. Of course, mortality rates are more appropriate if the goal is to reduce mortality among populations where screening programs can identify early stages of diseases, e.g., breast cancer or HIV infection, or where public health programs can reduce the mortality risk for other conditions, e.g., sudden infant death syndrome or alcohol-related motor vehicle accidents.

Using Intermediate Measures

Although incidence or mortality rates can be used to evaluate the effectiveness of public health programs, it may not be feasible to wait years to see these effects. Instead, the focus should be on identifying and using intermediate measures as long as there is sufficient Type I evidence supporting the relationship between changes in behavior and disease reduction in target populations. If the goal is to reduce breast cancer mortality, then an appropriate intermediate measure is the percentage of women 50 years of age or older who are screened annually for breast cancer. There is sufficient Type I evidence to show that mammography screening reduces the risk of breast cancer mortality among women 50–69 years of age.[2-7] Hence, programs designed to increase annual mammography screening rates in a community should reduce breast cancer mortality rates long-term by providing women, screened and diagnosed with early-stage breast cancer, with more effective treatment options. Other examples of intermediate measures are the percentage of residents in a community who choose not to smoke cigarettes (to reduce lung cancer risk), who exercise regularly (to reduce cardiovascular disease risk), or who practice safer sex (to reduce HIV infection risk). Furthermore, such measures, as changes in knowledge, attitudes, or intentions to change behavior may be very useful for determining the perceived health risk in the general population and whether perceptions differ within subgroups of the population.

Intermediate measures are not readily available for many populations. However, a data source that contains intermediate measures is the Behavioral Risk Factor Surveillance System (BRFSS), which provides prevalence data for health behaviors at a national and state level.[8] The rates are based on random samples of residents from each state who complete telephone-based questionnaires each year. For example, we know from this survey that 65% of Missouri women 50 years of age or older reported having a mammogram within the past year among those interviewed during 1999. This percentage alone, or combined with that of subsequent years, can be used to establish a baseline rate and to monitor the frequency of annual mammography screening for any new public health program designed to increase annual mammography screening rates in this population.

Estimating Disease Frequency for Smaller Populations

Disease rates can be estimated if all cases of disease can be enumerated for the population at risk during a specified period and the size of the population at risk (or amount of person-time) can be determined. In many countries, disease rates are routinely computed using birth and death certificate data since existing surveillance systems provide complete enumeration of these events. Although disease rates are commonly computed using national and state data, estimating similar rates for smaller geographically or demographically defined populations may be problematic. The main concern is the reliability of disease rates when there are too few cases of disease occurring in the population. As an example, the U.S. National Center for Health Statistics will not publish or release rates based on fewer than twenty observations. The reason behind this practice can be illustrated by examining the relative standard error based on various sample sizes, with rates based on fewer than twenty cases or deaths being very unreliable (Figure 5–1). The relative standard error is the standard error as a percentage of the measure itself.

A simple and sometimes effective solution is to expand the study (or observation) period by using multiple years to increase the number of cases of disease and person-time units for the target population. Another solution is to expand the population at risk by combining neighboring geographical areas or demographic groups, e.g., all ages or all races. Sometimes, "synthetic" estimates are useful. These estimates can be generated by using rates from larger geographic regions to estimate the number of cases of disease for smaller populations. For

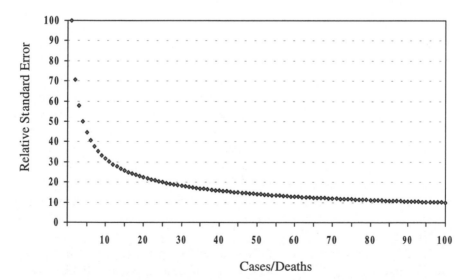

FIGURE 5–1. Relative standard error of an incidence or mortality rate as a function of the number of cases or deaths (*Source*: New York State Department of Health).

example, the number of cigarette smokers in a particular county can be estimated by multiplying the statewide smoking rate and the number of persons residing in the county. The Centers for Disease Control and Prevention (CDC) uses this approach in its smoking-attributable morbidity, mortality, and economic costs (SAMMEC) calculations.[9, 10]

Rosen and colleagues have provided guidance for analyzing regional data that take into account seven factors.[11] The factors include (1) when available, the importance of the health problem for a community; (2) the regional pattern of the descriptive data; (3) the (tested or anticipated) quality of the data; (4) the consistency of the data with other health indicators; (5) the consistency of the data with known risk factors; (6) trends in the data; and (7) the consistency of the data with other independent studies and with the experiences of local health personnel. Using these guidelines, they were able to show that alcohol-related mortality among men in a specific county in Sweden was lower but increasing faster than the national rate. Their step-by-step analysis dealt with many problems that are crucial in regional health analysis by looking closely at the quality of the data for their analysis and by examining trends using other factors associated with alcohol-related mortality.

CHARACTERIZING THE ISSUE BY PERSON, PLACE, AND TIME

Stratifying Rates by Person

Rates are routinely computed for specific diseases using data from public health surveillance systems. These rates, if computed for the total population, e.g., state or county populations, are crude (or unadjusted) rates since they represent the actual frequency of disease in the defined population for a specified period. Category-specific rates, which are "crude rates" for subgroups of the defined population, provide more information than crude rates about the patterns of disease. Category-specific rates are commonly used to characterize disease frequency by person, place, and time for a defined population (see example in Box 5–1). In most public health surveillance systems, demographic variables, e.g., age, sex, and race/ethnicity, are routinely collected for all members of the defined population. Some surveillance systems, e.g., BRFSS, also collect other demographic characteristics, including years of formal education, income level, and health insurance status.

Using category-specific rates to look at disease patterns will identify subgroups within the population with the highest disease rates and will allow us to hypothesize why the rates may be higher for some subgroups. For example,

Box 5–1. Suicide Rates by Person, Place, and Time

In 1998, suicide was the eighth leading cause of death in the United States. There were almost twice as many deaths due to suicide as homicide (30,575 versus 17,893 deaths). Overall, the crude suicide rate was 11.3 deaths per 100,000 population. Suicide rates by person, place, and time revealed the following trends:

- Suicide rates increase with age and are highest for people who are 80 years and older (21.0/100,000).
- Age-adjusted suicide rates are almost five times higher for males (19.3/100,000) than females (4.3/100,000), although females are more likely to attempt suicide.
- Age-adjusted suicide rates for native (12.6/100,000) and white Americans (12.2/100,000) are twice as high than other race/ethnic groups.
- Age-adjusted suicide rates are generally higher in the western states and lower in the eastern and midwestern states compared to the national rate.
- Age-adjusted suicide rates have been declining sporadically during the past 50 years from 13.2 deaths per 100,000 in 1950 to 11.3 deaths per 100,000 population in 1998.
- Nearly 3 of every 5 suicides are committed with a firearm.

breast cancer incidence and mortality rates by race/ethnicity, as shown in Figure 5–2, show fewer cases, but more deaths, for African American women. This discrepancy is partially because African American women are currently less likely to be screened annually for breast cancer and, in turn, are less likely to be diagnosed with local (or early stage) breast cancer. However, looking at mammography screening rates by income level from the BRFSS shows that the least-screened population is low-income women. If breast cancer mortality rates can be stratified by race/ethnicity and income level, we can determine if the highest mortality rate occurs among low-income women, women of color, or both subgroups. This additional information will allow us to identify high-risk groups that can be targeted with new public health programs designed to reduce the breast cancer burden in this population.

Stratifying Rates by Place

Category-specific rates are often computed to show patterns of disease by place of residence for the defined population. This information is routinely collected in most public health surveillance systems, and can be used to identify areas with the highest disease rates. Figure 5–3 shows breast cancer mortality rates by county, data that provide useful information for determining whether to implement new breast cancer mortality reduction programs in those counties where

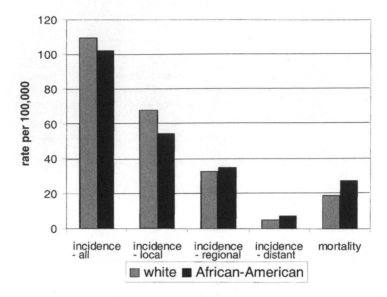

FIGURE 5–2. Age-adjusted breast cancer incidence and mortality rates by race for Missouri women, 1996–1998.

the mortality rates are highest rather than statewide. For larger metropolitan areas, zip codes, census tracts, and neighborhoods can be used to stratify disease rates geographically if the number of diseased persons and the size of the defined population are large enough to provide precise rates. This may provide additional information to pinpoint areas where HIV infection, homicide, or infant mortality rates are highest for a community. Other important variables, e.g., population density and migration patterns, can also be used to stratify disease rates, but are not usually collected in public health surveillance systems.

Stratifying Rates by Time

Category-specific rates, based on data from public health surveillance systems, are routinely reported each year. Looking at rates over time may reveal significant changes that have occurred in the population as the result of public health programs, changes in healthcare policies, or other events. Figure 5–4 shows breast cancer incidence and mortality rates for white and African American women in the United States for 1973–1998. In this example, the increase in breast cancer incidence rates during the 1980s is most likely due to a higher proportion of women who were being screened for breast cancer.[12, 13] It also shows that breast cancer incidence rates have been relatively stable for both groups of women since the early 1990s and that mortality rates are declining.

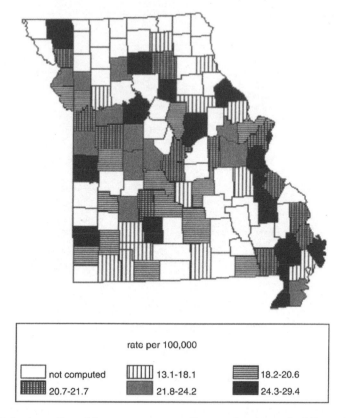

FIGURE 5–3. Age-adjusted breast cancer mortality rates by county for Missouri women, 1990–1998.

Although not often computed, disease rates by birth cohort are another way of looking at patterns of disease over time. In Figure 5–5, the lung cancer mortality rate for all men in the United States during 1998 (shown as the solid line in the figure) appears to increase with age, except for those 85 years of age or older. However, age-specific lung cancer mortality rates are higher for younger birth cohorts. For example, the lung cancer mortality rate for 65–74 year-old men is approximately 100 deaths per 100,000 men for those born between 1904 and 1895. The mortality rate for the same age group continues to increase in subsequent birth cohorts, with the highest rate of approximately 430 deaths per 100,000 for the cohort born between 1925 and 1934. The most logical explanation for this pattern is the differences in cumulative lifetime exposure to cigarette smoke seen in the birth cohorts that are represented in this population during 1998. In other words, members of the population born after 1905 were more likely to smoke cigarettes and to smoke for longer periods than those born

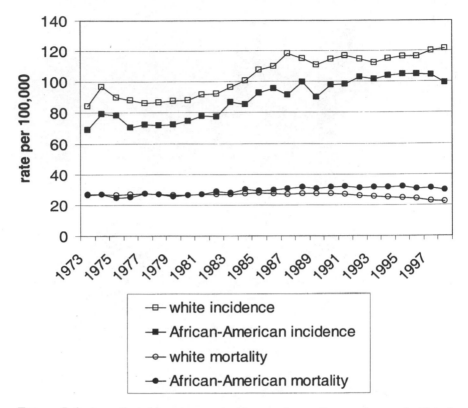

FIGURE 5–4. Age-adjusted breast cancer incidence and mortality rates by year for United States women, 1973–1998. Incidence rates based on data from nine cancer registries of the Cancer Surveillance, Epidemiology, and End Results (SEER) program.

prior to 1905. Hence, the increasing age-specific lung cancer mortality rates reflect the increasing prevalence of cigarette smokers in the population for subsequent birth cohorts.

Adjusting Rates

Although category-specific rates are commonly used to characterize patterns of disease for defined populations, it is sometimes necessary to adjust rates. Crude rates are often adjusted when the objective is to compare the disease rates between populations or within the same population over time. Rate adjustment is a technique for "removing" the effects of age (or any other factor) from crude rates so as to allow meaningful comparisons across populations with different age structures or distributions. For example, comparing the crude lung cancer mortality rate in Florida (78 deaths per 100,000 persons) to that of Alaska (31

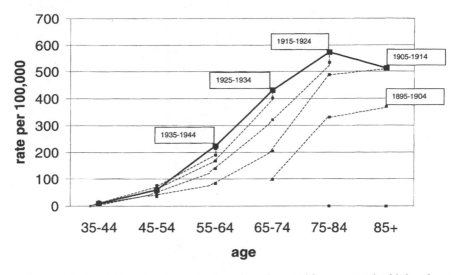

FIGURE 5–5. Mortality rates due to trachea, bronchus, and lung cancer by birth cohort for United States men. Heavy line represents age-specific mortality rates for 1998. Dashed lines represent age-specific rates for birth cohorts denoted by labels in boxes.

deaths per 100,000 persons) is misleading, since the relatively older population in Florida will lead to a higher crude death rate, even if the age-specific lung cancer mortality rates in Florida and Alaska are similar. For such a comparison, age-adjusted rates are preferable.

The calculations required to compute age-adjusted rates are fairly straight forward, as shown in Table 5–1. First, age-specific lung cancer mortality rates are generated for each state. Second, the age-specific lung cancer mortality rates for each state are multiplied times the number of persons in the corresponding age groups from the 2000 United States standard population (which have been prorated to equal 1,000,000). This produces the number of "expected" deaths in each age group if the numbers of persons at risk of dying in each age group were the same for the state and United States populations. The total number of expected deaths in each state is then divided by the total number of persons in the United States standard population to compute the age-adjusted lung cancer mortality rate for Florida (60 deaths per 100,000) and Alaska (58 deaths per 100,000) residents.

PUBLIC HEALTH SURVEILLANCE SYSTEMS

Public health surveillance is the ongoing collection and timely analysis, interpretation, and communication of health information for public health action.

Table 5–1. Direct Adjustment of Lung Cancer Mortality Rates for Florida and Utah Residents (1996–1998)

Age (years)	FLORIDA			ALASKA		
	Lung Cancer Mortality Rate/ 100,000	2000 Standard U.S. Population	Expected Number of Deaths	Lung Cancer Mortality Rate/ 100,000	2000 Standard U.S. Population	Expected Number of Deaths
<5	0.00	110,589	0.00	0.00	110,589	0.00
5–14	0.00	145,565	0.00	0.00	145,565	0.00
15–24	0.04	138,646	0.06	0.00	138,646	0.00
25–34	0.86	135,573	1.17	0.42	135,573	0.57
35–44	8.19	162,613	13.32	5.58	162,613	9.07
45–54	43.07	134,834	58.07	27.75	134,834	37.42
55–64	145.81	87,247	127.21	107.54	87,247	93.83
65–74	282.21	66,037	186.36	361.77	66,037	238.90
75–84	359.08	44,842	161.02	383.77	44,842	172.09
85+	344.10	15,508	53.36	187.03	15,508	29.00
Total		1,000,000	600.57		1,000,000	580.88

Age-adjusted lung cancer mortality rate for Florida residents
= 600.57 deaths/1,000,000 persons
= 60 deaths/100,000 persons

Age-adjusted lung cancer mortality rate for Alaska residents
= 580.88 deaths/1,000,000 persons
= 58 deaths/100,000 persons

Public health surveillance systems are maintained at federal, state, and local levels, and can be used to estimate the frequency of diseases and other health conditions for defined populations. At least five major purposes for surveillance systems can be described: (1) assessing health and monitoring health status and health risks; (2) following disease-specific events and trends; (3) planning, implementing, monitoring, and evaluating health programs and policies; (4) conducting financial management and monitoring information; and (5) conducting public health research.[14] The few surveillance systems that currently exist can provide information on births, deaths, infectious diseases, cancers, birth defects, and health behaviors. Each system usually contains sufficient information to estimate prevalence or incidence rates and to describe the frequency of diseases or health condition by person, place, and time. Although data from surveillance systems can be used to obtain baseline and follow-up measurements for target populations, there may be limitations when using the data to evaluate intervention effectiveness for narrowly defined populations. In this case, it may be necessary to estimate the frequency of disease or other health condition for the target population by using special surveys or one of the study designs described later in this chapter.

Vital Statistics

Vital statistics are based on data from birth and death certificates and are used to monitor disease patterns within and across defined populations. Birth certificates include information about maternal/paternal/newborn demographics, lifestyle exposures during pregnancy, medical history, obstetric procedures, and labor/delivery complications for all live births. Fetal death certificates include the same data, in addition to the cause of death, for all fetal deaths that exceed a minimum gestational age and/or birth weight. The data collected on birth and fetal death certificates are similar for many states and territories since the design of the certificates were modified, based on standard federal recommendations issued in 1989. The reliability of the data has also improved since changing from a "write in" to a "check box" format, although some variables are more reliable than others.[15–17] Additional improvements are expected once new standard federal recommendations are implemented in 2003 or later. Birth-related outcomes—maternal smoking, preterm delivery, and fetal death rates—are routinely monitored, using data from birth and fetal death certificates.

Like birth certificates, death certificates provide complete enumeration of all events in a defined population. Death certificates include demographic and cause-of-death data that are used to compute disease- and injury-specific mortality rates. Mortality rates can be estimated for local populations if the number of deaths and the size of the defined population are large enough to provide precise rates. Birth and death certificates are generated locally and maintained at state health departments. Data from birth and death certificates are analyzed at state and national levels and electronically stored at state health departments and the National Center for Health Statistics.

Reportable Diseases

In addition to vital statistics, all states and territories mandate the reporting of some diseases. Although the type of reportable diseases may differ by state or territory, they usually include specific childhood, foodborne, sexually transmitted, and other infectious diseases. These diseases are reported by physicians and other health care providers to local public health authorities and are monitored for early signs of epidemics in the community. The data are maintained by local and state health departments and are submitted weekly to the CDC for national surveillance and reporting. Disease frequencies are stratified by age, gender, race/ethnicity, and place of residence, and reported routinely in the *Morbidity and Mortality Weekly Report (MMWR)*. However, reporting is influenced by disease severity, availability of public health measures, public concern, ease of reporting, and physician appreciation of public health practice in the community.[18]

Registries

Disease registries routinely monitor defined populations, thereby providing very reliable estimates of disease frequency. All fifty states have active cancer registries supported by the state or federal government. These registries provide data that can be used to compute site-specific cancer incidence rates for a community, if the number of cancers and the size of the defined population are large enough to provide precise rates. Since 1973, the federally sponsored Cancer Surveillance, Epidemiology and End Results (SEER) program has provided estimates of national cancer rates based on 10%–15% of the total population.[19] Along with state-based cancer registries, this surveillance system can provide rates for specific types of cancer, characterized by person, place, and time. All invasive cancers that occur among the state's residents are confirmed pathologically and recorded electronically for surveillance and research purposes. They are also linked with death certificates to provide additional information about disease-specific survival rates.

In 1998, the U.S. Congress passed the Birth Defects Prevention Act that authorized CDC to collect, analyze, and make available data on birth defects; operate regional centers for applied epidemiologic research on the prevention of birth defects; and inform and educate the public about the prevention of birth defects. Subsequently, CDC awarded cooperative agreements to specific states to address major problems that hinder the surveillance of birth defects and the use of data for prevention and intervention programs. The states were awarded funding to initiate new surveillance systems where none now exist, to support new systems, or to improve existing surveillance systems. Birth defects registries are either active or passive reporting surveillance systems designed to identify birth defects diagnosed for all stillborn and live-born infants. Active reporting surveillance systems provide more reliable estimates of the prevalence of specific birth defects, if staff and resources are available to search medical records from hospitals, laboratories, and other medical sources for all diagnosed birth defects in a defined population. Passive reporting surveillance systems are designed to estimate the prevalence of birth defects that can be identified using computer algorithms to link and search birth certificates, death certificates, patient abstract systems, and other readily available electronic databases.

Surveys

There are several federally sponsored surveys, including the National Health Interview Survey (NHIS), National Health and Nutrition Examination Survey (NHANES), and BRFSS, that have been designed to monitor the nation's health. These surveys are designed to measure numerous health indices, including acute and chronic diseases, injuries, disabilities, and other health-related outcomes. Some surveys are ongoing annual surveillance systems, while others are conducted periodically. These surveys usually provide prevalence estimates for specific diseases among adults and children in the United States. Although the surveys can also provide prevalence estimates for regions and individual states, they cannot currently be used to produce estimates for smaller geographically defined populations.

USE OF THE INTERNET AND OTHER READILY AVAILABLE TOOLS

Some data sources and tools are readily available on the Internet and can be used to estimate baseline and follow-up rates for needs assessment and for evaluating the effectiveness of new public health interventions. The data from some national and state-based public health surveillance systems can be obtained online or from reports from websites maintained by the sponsoring agencies. An array of state and territory health departments and other governmental and agency websites can be accessed from the CDC website <http://www.cdc.gov/other.htm>.

Some websites contain interactive, point-and-click menus that can be used to generate customized reports of crude, category-specific, and adjusted rates for defined populations. Three interactive programs (CDC WONDER, WISQARS, and BRFSS) from the CDC web site are examples. CDC WONDER <http://wonder.cdc.gov> is an easy-to-use system that provides a wide variety of reports (including the *MMWR*) and prevention guidelines. It allows the user to query numerous public health surveillance systems, which provide natality, mortality and other types of data. It can provide disease rates by age, gender, and race/ethnicity for the nation and individual states and counties. WISQARS (Web-based Injury Statistics Query and Reporting System) <http://www.cdc.gov/ncipc/wisqars> is an interactive system that provides injury-related mortality data. WISQRS can be used to estimate mortality rates for specific external causes of injuries for the nation and individual states. It can also be used to generate reports showing injury-specific mortality rates by mechanism/cause or manner/intent by age, gender, and race/ethnicity. The BRFSS <http://www.cdc.gov/nccdphp/brfss> provides national and state-specific estimates of health behaviors related to health care access, immunization, diet, weight control, physical activity, sexual behavior, use of tobacco, alcohol, and firearms, cholesterol and hypertension awareness, screening for breast, cervical, colorectal, and prostate cancer, and prevalence of arthritis, asthma, cardiovascular disease, diabetes, HIV, and oral health. Similar information is also now available for larger metropolitan areas or regions within states. An interactive menu can be used to generate prevalence and trend data for any of the questions asked in the annual survey by age, gender, race/ethnicity, education, and income level.

A few states currently have their own interactive, web-based system for generating rates from their public health surveillance systems. One example is the Missouri Information for Community Assessment (MICA) <http://www.dhss.state.mo.us/MICA/nojava.html>. Like the interactive menus found in CDC WONDER, MICA is an interactive system that allows the user to compute rates based on birth, death, and hospital discharge data. As shown in Figure 5–6, category-specific death rates can be stratified by age, gender, race/ethnicity, county of residence, and year of occurrence. The rates can be displayed in reports or maps with counties/cities shaded according to user-defined criteria. The data can also be downloaded for use in other applications, e.g., Microsoft Excel, to produce additional charts or graphs.

The Community Health Status Indicators (CHSI) Project <http://www.communityhealth.hrsa.gov> was launched in response to grassroots requests from local health officials for health data at the local level. The Health Resources and Services Administration sponsored and funded the project through collaboration among the Association of State and Territorial Health Officials, the National Association of County and City Health Officials, and the Public Health

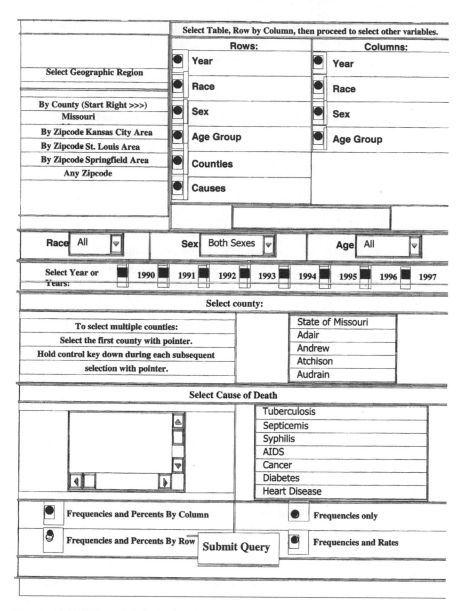

FIGURE 5–6. Missouri Information for Community Assessment (MICA) menu.

Foundation. From this collaborative, the CHSI report emerged in a unique, easy-to-use format. The CHSI report provides a profile of each county's overall health status, using a broad spectrum of health indicators. Counties can compare their health indicators to *Healthy People 2010* targets, national rates, and other peer counties that are similar in characteristics, e.g., population size, density, age distribution, and poverty. For health officials currently working in jurisdictions lacking the infrastructure to collect data, the CHSI reports can serve as a tool for targeting resources and setting priorities.

BASIC OVERVIEW OF ANALYTIC EPIDEMIOLOGY

As stated earlier, descriptive epidemiology provides information about the patterns of disease within defined populations that can be used to generate etiologic or intervention-based hypotheses. These hypotheses can be evaluated using study designs and analytic methods that encompass the principles of analytic epidemiology. Most study designs can be used to provide Type I evidence to support causal associations between modifiable (and nonmodifiable) risk factors and specific diseases. Once there is sufficient Type I evidence, additional work is needed to determine the effectiveness of public health programs designed to reduce the prevalence of these risk factors in the population. Experimental and quasi-experimental study designs are generally used, depending upon available resources and timing, to evaluate the effectiveness of new public health programs. Issues related to program and policy evaluation are also covered in Chapter 9.

Experimental Study Designs

Experimental study designs provide the most convincing evidence that new public health programs are effective. If study participants are randomized into groups (or arms), the study design is commonly called a randomized controlled trial. When two groups are created, the study participants allocated randomly to one group are given the new intervention (or treatment) and those allocated to the other group serve as controls. The study participants in both groups are followed prospectively, and disease (or health-related outcome) rates are computed for each group at the end of the observation period. Since both groups are identical in all aspects, except for the intervention, a lower disease rate in the intervention group implies that the intervention is effective.

The same study design can also be used to randomize groups instead of individuals to evaluate the effectiveness of health behavior interventions for communities. Referred to as a group-randomized trial, groups of study participants, e.g., schools within a school system or communities within a state, are randomized to receive the intervention or to serve as controls for the study. Initially, the groups may be paired, based on similar characteristics. Then, each group within each pair is allocated randomly to the intervention or control group. This helps to balance the distribution of characteristics of the study participants for both study groups and to reduce potential study bias. The intervention is applied to all individuals in the intervention group, and withheld or delayed for the control group. Measurements are taken at baseline and at the end of the observation period to determine if there are significant differences between the disease rates for the intervention and control groups. Both experimental study designs have been used to evaluate the effectiveness of public health interventions designed to increase immunization coverage[20, 21] and physical activity[22] in target populations, as examples.

Quasi-Experimental Study Designs

Experimental study designs are considered the gold standard, since randomization of study participants reduces the potential for study bias. However, it is not always feasible to use this study design when evaluating new public health programs. Often, quasi-experimental study designs are used to evaluate the effectiveness of new programs. Quasi-experimental studies are identical in design to experimental studies, except that the study participants are not allocated randomly to the intervention or control group. Study participants allocated to both groups are followed for a predetermined period, and disease rates are computed for each group to determine if the intervention is effective. As is the case for experimental study designs, baseline (or pre-intervention) measurements are crucial since the investigator must determine how similar the intervention and control groups are prior to the intervention. Ideally, disease rates should be identical at baseline and for the period prior to the execution of the study. Examining the characteristics of the study groups by person, place, and time will reduce the probability of concluding that the intervention is effective when actually there are other factors historically affecting the disease rate in the community.

If a comparable control group is not available, quasi-experimental study designs can still be used to measure the impact of public health interventions on a particular health outcome in the same population. Actually, quasi-experimental study designs are commonly used when comparing new public health initiatives that affect the total population. Some examples are the impact of new state laws requiring the use of seat belts[23] and child safety seats[24] or laws enacted to reduce alcohol-impaired driving.[25] In this study design, the population must be observed for a period prior to the intervention to show that the disease rate was stable before the intervention is implemented. Study designs that analyze disease rates or trends over time before and after implementing the new intervention are sometimes referred to as time-series studies (see example in Box 5–2 and Figure 5–7). It is also prudent to measure the prevalence of related risk factors in the population to determine if the risk factors are stable during the study period. Since there is no external control group, additional information describing the population before and after the implementation of the new intervention can be

Box 5–2. *Back to Sleep* Campaign

Before 1992 there was mounting epidemiologic evidence from around the world that infants placed in the prone sleeping position were at increased risk of sudden infant death syndrome (SIDS).[30–39] Other potential risk factors were soft bedding, swaddling, and recent respiratory or gastrointestinal illnesses. In 1992, the American Academy of Pediatrics (AAP) recommended placing healthy infants on their sides or backs rather than their abdomens.[40] They also recommended removing soft surfaces or objects from the infant's sleeping environment that might trap exhaled air. These recommendations led to a nationwide public health intervention, referred to as the *Back to Sleep* campaign and implemented in 1994, which was designed to educate all parents, grandparents, and health care professionals. The national goal of the *Back to Sleep* campaign was to reduce the percentage of infants put to sleep on their abdomens to 10 percent or less by the year 2000. Since implementing this program, the prevalence of infants sleeping in the prone position has decreased steadily from 70% in 1992 to 24% in 1996.[41] The SIDS rates (shown in Figure 5–7) reflect the changes in infant sleep position for the same period, using a quasi-experimental study design and time series analysis. Overall, SIDS rates have decreased from 1.3 deaths per 1,000 live births in 1990 to 0.7 deaths per 1,000 live births in 1998. However, African American and native American infants are still 2.4 to 2.8 times more likely to die of SIDS than white infants.[42] As a result of these findings, focus groups were conducted to examine why certain populations were not hearing the *Back to Sleep* message in order to develop more effective intervention strategies for these high-risk groups.

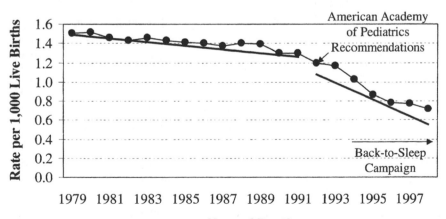

FIGURE 5–7. Time-series analysis of U.S. sudden infant death syndrome (SIDS) rates, 1989–1995.

used to strengthen the conclusions regarding the effectiveness of the new intervention.

Observational Study Designs

Since it may not be ethical to use experimental or quasi-experimental study designs in all research settings, investigators can use observational study designs to evaluate hypotheses that prior exposures increase the risk of specific diseases. Generally, observational study designs are used to provide Type I evidence, for which the exposure has already occurred and disease patterns can be studied for those with and without the exposure of interest. A good historical example is the association between cigarette use and lung cancer. Since people choose whether or not to smoke cigarettes, we can evaluate the hypothesis that cigarette smokers are at increased risk of developing lung cancer by following smokers and non-smokers over time to assess their lung cancer rates.

Cohort and case-control studies are two observational study designs that can be used to evaluate the strength of the association between prior exposure and risk of disease in the study population. Cohort studies compare the disease rates of exposed and unexposed study participants who are disease-free at baseline and followed over time to estimate the disease rates in both groups. Cohort studies are often conducted when the exposure of interest is rare in the community, since all who have been exposed can be identified and followed to determine if the disease rate is significantly higher (or lower) than the rates for unexposed individuals from the same population. Studies that have focused on the effects of diet or exercise on specific diseases or health-related outcomes[26] are good examples of cohort studies.

Case-control studies compare the frequency of prior exposures for study participants who have been diagnosed recently with the disease (cases) with those who have not developed the disease (controls). Case-control studies are the preferred study design when the disease is rare, and they are efficient when studying diseases with long latency. As is true for all study designs, selecting appropriate controls and obtaining reliable exposure estimates are crucial when evaluating any hypothesis that a prior exposure increases (or decreases) the risk of a specific disease.[27, 28]

Cross-sectional studies, a third type of observational study designs, can be completed relatively quickly and inexpensively to look at associations between exposure and disease. Since information regarding potential exposures and existing diseases for the study participants is measured simultaneously when the study is conducted, cross-sectional studies are unable to ascertain whether the exposure preceded the development of the disease among the study participants. Hence, cross-sectional studies are used primarily to generate hypotheses. Nevertheless, cross-sectional studies are used for public health planning and evaluation. For example, if a public health administrator wants to know how many women of reproductive age smoked cigarettes while pregnant, knowledge about the prevalence of maternal smoking in the community is important. Knowing the maternal smoking rates for subgroups of this population will help target interventions, if needed, for each subgroup. Cross-sectional studies are also used to help set research priorities based on consideration of the disease burden. For example, a study of the prevalence of chronic gynecologic conditions among United States women of reproductive age found that the most common conditions are menstrual disorders, adnexal condition, and uterine fibroids. This information suggests that not only are more effective treatments for these disorders needed, but also that more research on their causation is desirable.[29]

SUMMARY

As they develop, implement, and evaluate new public health intervention programs, public health professionals need basic epidemiologic skills in order to quantify the frequency of disease in target populations.

Essential points from this chapter include the following:

- Knowing the frequency of disease in the population before implementing any new public health program is crucial, and can help focus efforts for reducing the disease burden by targeting high-risk groups in the population.
- Public health surveillance systems provide the necessary data to measure the frequency of some diseases, but special surveys are often needed to obtain baseline data for other diseases in defined populations.
- Public health surveillance data are currently available via the Internet for some diseases and can be used to look interactively at disease patterns by person, place, and time.
- Understanding how epidemiology studies are designed will improve how we evaluate existing data when determining the likelihood of new causal associations and effective public health programs for reducing the disease burden.

SUGGESTED READINGS AND WEBSITES

Readings

Brownson RC, Petitti DB. *Applied Epidemiology: Theory to Practice.* New York: Oxford University Press, 1998.

Cook TD, Campbell DT. *Quasi-Experimentation: Design and Analysis Issues for Field Settings.* Boston: Houghton Mifflin, 1979.

Friis HF, Sellers TA. *Epidemiology for Public Health Practice*. 2nd ed. Gaithersburg, Maryland: Aspen Publishers, Inc, 1999.

Gordis L. *Epidemiology*. Philadelphia: W.B. Saunders Company, 1996.

Kelsey JL Whittemore AS, Evans AS. *Methods in Observational Epidemiology*. 2nd ed. New York: Oxford University Press, 1996.

Meinert CL. *Clinical Trials: Design, Conduct, and Analysis*. New York: Oxford University Press, 1985.

Murray DM. *Design and Analysis of Group-Randomized Trials*. New York: Oxford University Press, 1998.

Rothman KJ, Greenland S. *Modern Epidemiology*. 2nd ed. Philadelphia: Lippincott-Raven Publishers, 1998.

Teutsch SM, Churchill RE, eds. *Principles and Practice of Public Health Surveillance*. 2nd ed. New York: Oxford University Press, 2000.

Selected Websites

CDC BRFSS <http://www.cdc.gov/nccdphp/brfss> The BRFSS, an ongoing data collection program conducted in all states, the District of Columbia, and three U.S. territories, and the world's largest telephone survey, tracks health risks in the United States. Information from the survey is used to improve the health of the American people. The CDC has developed a standard core questionnaire so that data can be compared across various strata.

CDC WONDER <http://wonder.cdc.gov> CDC WONDER is an easy-to-use system that provides a single point of access to a wide variety of CDC reports, guidelines, and numeric public health data. It can be valuable in public health research, decision making, priority setting, program evaluation, and resource allocation.

National Center for Health Statistics <http://www.cdc.gov/nchs/> National Center for Health Statistics is the principal vital and health statistics agency for the U.S. government. NCHS data systems include information on vital events as well as information on health status, lifestyle and exposure to unhealthy influences, the onset and diagnosis of illness and disability, and the use of health care. NCHS has two major types of data systems: systems based on populations, containing data collected through personal interviews or examinations, e.g., National Health Interview Survey and National Health and Nutrition Examination Survey and systems based on records, containing data collected from vital and medical records. These data are used by policymakers in Congress and the administration, by medical researchers, and by others in the health community.

Epidemiology Supercourse <http://www.pitt.edu/~super1/> This course coordinated by the University of Pittsburgh School of Public Health, is designed to provide an overview on epidemiology and the Internet for medical and health-freedom related students around the world.

Kansas Information for Communities <http://kic.kdhe.state.ks.us/kic/> The Kansas Information for Communities (KIC) system gives data users the chance to prepare their own queries for vital-event and other health-care data. The queries designed into this system can answer many health data requests. As KIC is implemented, more data will be added. KIC programs will allow users to generate their own tables for specific characteristics, year of occurrence, age, rate, sex, and county.

Missouri Information for Community Assessment <http://www.dhss.state.mo.us/MICA/nojava.html> The Missouri Information for Community Assessment (MICA) system is an interactive system that allows anyone to create a table of specific data from various data files including births, deaths, hospital discharges and others. The user can also produce a map with counties and/or cities shaded according to user-defined criteria.

Texas Health Data <http://soupfin.tdh.state.tx.us/> Texas Health Data allows a user to generate a table showing frequencies, frequencies and rates, frequencies and percents by column or row, and a map showing frequencies or frequencies and rates by quartiles or quintiles. At present, the years of data available for births are 1990 through 1999. Population estimates and projections are available for 1990 through 2010.

REFERENCES

1. Terris M. The Society for Epidemiologic Research (SER) and the future of epidemiology. American Journal of Epidemiology 1992;136(8):909–915.
2. Shapiro S, Venet W, Strax P. *Periodic screening for breast cancer: The Health Insurance Plan project and its sequelae, 1963–1986.* Baltimore Johns Hopkins University Press, 1988.
3. Roberts MM, Alexander FE, Anderson TJ, et al. Edinburgh trial of screening for breast cancer: Mortality at seven years. *Lancet* 1990;335(8684):241–246.
4. Frisell J, Eklund G, Hellstrom L, Lidbrink E, Rutqvist LE, Somell A. Randomized study of mammography screening—preliminary report on mortality in the Stockholm trial. *Breast Cancer Research and Treatment* 1991;18(1):49–56.
5. Tabar L, Fagerberg G, Duffy SW, Day NE, Gad A, Grontoft O. Update of the Swedish two-county program of mammographic screening for breast cancer. *Radiology Clinics of North America* 1992;30(1):187–210.
6. Miller AB, Baines CJ, To T, Wall C. Canadian National Breast Screening Study: 2. Breast cancer detection and death rates among women aged 50 to 59 years. *Canadian Medical Association Journal* 1992;147(10):1477–1488.
7. Nystrom L, Rutqvist LE, Wall S, et al. Breast cancer screening with mammography: overview of Swedish randomised trials. *Lancet* 1993;341(8851):973–978.
8. Siegel PZ, Brackbill RM, Frazier EL, et al. Behavioral risk factor surveillance, 1986–1990. *Morbidity and Mortality Weekly Report* 1991;40:1–23.
9. Shultz JM, Novotny TE, Rice DP. Quantifying the disease impact of cigarette smoking with SAMMEC II software. *Public Health Representative.* 1991;106(3):326–333.
10. Nelson DE, Kirkendall RS, Lawton RL, et al. Surveillance for smoking—attributable mortality and years of potential life lost, by state—United States, 1990. *Morbidity and Mortality Weekly Report Surveillance Summaries* 1994;43(1):1–8.
11. Rosen M, Nystrom L, Wall S. Guidelines for regional mortality analysis: an epidemiological approach to health planning. *International Journal of Epidemiology* 1985; 14(2):293–299.
12. Chu KC, Tarone RE, Kessler LG, et al. Recent trends in U.S. breast cancer incidence, survival, and mortality rates. *Journal of the National Cancer Institute* 1996;88(21): 1571–1579.
13. Chevarley F, White E. Recent trends in breast cancer mortality among white and black U.S. women. *American Journal of Public Health* 1997;87(5):775–781.
14. White ME, McDonnell SM. Public health surveillance in low- and middle-income countries. In: Teutsch SM and Churchill RE, eds. *Principles and Practice of Public Health Surveillance.* 2nd ed. New York: Oxford University Press; 2000, pp. 287–315.

15. Frost F, Starzyk P, George S, McLaughlin JF. Birth complication reporting: The effect of birth certificate design. *American Journal of Public Health* 1984;74(5):505–506.
16. Buescher PA, Taylor KP, Davis MH, Bowling JM. The quality of the new birth certificate data: A validation study in North Carolina. *American Journal of Public Health* 1993;83(8):1163–1165.
17. Piper JM, Mitchel EFJ, Snowden M, Hall C, Adams M, Taylor P. Validation of 1989 Tennessee birth certificates using maternal and newborn hospital records. *American Journal of Epidemiology* 1993;137(7):758–768.
18. Thacker SB, Stroup DF. Future directions for comprehensive public health surveillance and health information systems in the United States. *American Journal of Epidemiology* 1994;140(5):383–397.
19. Gloeckler-Ries LA, Hankey BF, Edwards Bk, eds. *Cancer Statistics Review, 1973–1987*. NIH Publication No. 90–2789. Bethesda, MD: National Cancer Institute, 1990.
20. Shefer A, Briss P, Rodewald L, et al. Improving immunization coverage rates: an evidence-based review of the literature. *Epidemiology Reviews* 1999;21(1):96–142.
21. Briss PA, Rodewald LE, Hinman AR, et al. Reviews of evidence regarding interventions to improve vaccination coverage in children, adolescents, and adults. The Task Force on Community Preventive Services. *American Journal of Preventive Medicine* 2000;18(1 Suppl):97–140.
22. Task Force on Community Preventive Services. Increasing physical activity: a report on recommendations of the task force on community preventive services. *Morbidity and Mortality Weekly Report* October 26, 2001 2001;50(RR18):1–16.
23. Dinh-Zarr TB, Sleet DA, Shults RA, et al. Reviews of evidence regarding interventions to increase the use of safety belts. *American Journal of Preventive Medicine* 2001;21(4 Suppl 1):48–65.
24. Zaza S, Sleet DA, Thompson RS, Sosin DM, Bolen JC. Reviews of evidence regarding interventions to increase use of child safety seats. *American Journal of Preventive Medicine* 2001;21(4 Suppl 1):31–47.
25. Shults RA, Elder RW, Sleet DA, et al. Reviews of evidence regarding interventions to reduce alcohol-impaired driving. *American Journal of Preventive Medicine* 2001; 21(4 Suppl 1):66–88.
26. Hu FB, Manson JE, Stampfer MJ, et al. Diet, lifestyle, and the risk of type 2 diabetes mellitus in women. *New England Journal of Medicine* 2001;345(11):790–797.
27. Thompson RS, Rivara FP, Thompson DC. A case-control study of the effectiveness of bicycle safety helmets. *New England Journal of Medicine* 1989;320(21):1361–1367.
28. White E, Malone KE, Weiss NS, Daling JR. Breast cancer among young U.S. women in relation to oral contraceptive use. *Journal of the National Cancer Institute* 1994; 86(7):505–514.
29. Kjerulff KH, Erickson BA, Langenberg PW. Chronic gynecological conditions reported by US women: findings from the National Health Interview Survey, 1984 to 1992. *American Journal of Public Health.* 1996;86(2):195–199.
30. Carpenter RG, Shaddick CW. Role of infection, suffocation, and bottle-feeding in cot death. *British Journal of Preventive and Social Medicine* 1965;19:1–7.
31. Frogatt P. Epidemiologic aspects of the Northern Ireland study. In: Bergman AS, Beckwith JB and Ray CG, eds. *Sudden Infant Death Syndrome*. Seattle: University of Washington Press, 1970, pp. 32–46.

32. Beal SM, Blundell H. Sudden infant death syndrome related to position in the cot. *Medical Journal of Australia* 1978;2(5):217–218.
33. de Jonge GA, Engelberts AC, Koomen-Liefting AJ, Kostense PJ. Cot death and prone sleeping position in The Netherlands. *British Medical Journal* 1989;298(6675):722.
34. McGlashan ND. Sudden infant deaths in Tasmania, 1980–1986: A seven year prospective study. *Social Science and Medicine* 1989;29(8):1015–1026.
35. Lee NN, F. CY, Davies DP, Lau E, Yip DC. Sudden infant deaths in Hong Kong: Confirmation of low incidence. *British Medical Journal* 1989;298:721.
36. Fleming PJ, Gilbert R, Azaz Y, et al. Interaction between bedding and sleeping position in the sudden infant death syndrome: a population based case-control study. *British Medical Journal* 1990;301(6743):85–89.
37. Mitchell EA, Scragg R, Stewart AW, et al. Results from the first year of the New Zealand cot death study. *New Zealand Medical Journal* 1991;104(906):71–76.
38. Dwyer T, Ponsonby AL, Newman NM, Gibbons LE. Prospective cohort study of prone sleeping position and sudden infant death syndrome. *Lancet* 1991;337(8752): 1244–1247.
39. Dwyer T, Ponsonby AL, Gibbons LE, Newman NM. Prone sleeping position and SIDS: Evidence from recent case-control and cohort studies in Tasmania. *Journal of Paediatrics and Child Health* 1991;27(6):340–343.
40. Willinger M, Hoffman HJ, Hartford RB. Infant sleep position and risk for sudden infant death syndrome: Report of meeting held January 13 and 14, 1994, National Institutes of Health, Bethesda, MD. *Pediatrics* 1994;93(5):814–819.
41. Positioning and sudden infant death syndrome (SIDS): update. American Academy of Pediatrics Task Force on Infant Positioning and SIDS. *Pediatrics* 1996;98(6 Pt 1):1216–1218.
42. Centers for Disease Control and Prevention. Progress in reducing risky infant sleeping positions—13 states, 1996–1998. *Morbidity and Mortality Weekly Report* 1999; 48(39):878–882.

6

Searching the Scientific Literature and Organizing Information

> Where is the wisdom we have lost in knowledge? Where is the knowledge we have lost in information?
>
> —T.S. Eliot

As you develop an issue statement and begin to understand the epidemiologic nature of a particular public health issue along with the intervention options, the scientific literature is a crucial source of information. Because of the growth in the amount of information available to public health practitioners, it is essential to follow a systematic approach to literature searching. The underpinnings of an evidence-based process rest largely on one's ability to find credible, high-quality evidence as efficiently and exhaustively as possible. A systematic searching process also helps ensure that others can replicate the same results. Modern information technologies, in particular the increasing capacity of personal computers and the rapid growth of the Internet, provide an excellent opportunity to find valuable information quickly.

This chapter provides guidance on how to search the scientific literature. It focuses on the importance of a literature search, where to search, how to find evidence, and how to organize the results of a search. Evaluation of the quality of the evidence is covered in other chapters (primarily Chapters 1, 2, and 5).

BACKGROUND

As noted in Chapter 1, there are many types and sources of evidence on public health programs and policies. Scientific information (the "scientific literature") on theory and practice can be found in textbooks, government reports, scientific journals, policy statements, on the Internet, and at scientific meetings. Three levels of reading the scientific literature have been described: (1) browsing—

flicking through books and articles, looking for anything of interest; (2) reading for information—approaching the literature in search of an answer to a specific question; and (3) reading for research—reading in order to obtain a comprehensive view of the existing state of knowledge on a specific topic.[1] In practice, most of us obtain most of our information through browsing.[2] However, to conduct a literature review for building evidence-based programs efficiently, it is important to take a more structured approach. We focus primarily on journal publications here because they have gone through a process of peer review to enhance the quality of the information and are the closest thing to a gold standard that is available (see Chapter 2).

When conducting a search of the scientific literature, there are four types of publications to look for:

1. Original research articles: the papers written by the authors who conducted the research. These articles provide details on the methods used, results, and implications of results. A thorough and comprehensive summary of a body of literature will consist of careful reading of original research articles.
2. Review articles: a narrative summary of what is known on a particular topic. A review article presents a summary of original research articles. The *Annual Review of Public Health*[3] is an excellent source of review articles on a variety of topics. A limitation of review articles is that they do not always follow systematic approaches, a practice that sometimes leads to inconsistent results.[4]
3. Review articles featuring a quantitative synthesis of results: a quantitative synthesis involves a process such as meta-analysis—a quantitative approach that provides a systematic, organized, and structured way of integrating the findings of individual research studies.[5, 6] This type of review is often called a systematic review (Chapter 3). In meta-analysis, researchers produce a summary statistical estimate of the measure of association. For example, the Cochrane Collaboration, an international organization of clinicians, epidemiologists, and others, has produced quantitative reviews on the effectiveness of various health care interventions. <www.cochrane.org>
4. Guidelines: Practice guidelines are formal statements that offer advice to clinicians, public health practitioners, managed-care organizations, and the public on how to improve the effectiveness and impact of clinical and public health interventions. Guidelines translate the findings of research and demonstration projects into accessible and useable information for public health practice. There are several examples of useful guidelines.[7-10] The terminology used within them differs across the globe. Thus, in the European Community, directives are stronger than recommendations, which are stronger than guidelines.[11] No such hierarchy exists in North America.

Review articles and guidelines often present a useful short cut for many busy practitioners who do not have the time to master the literature on multiple public health topics.

In addition to the type of publication, timeliness of scientific information is an important consideration. To find the best quality evidence for medical decision making, Sackett and colleagues have recommended that practitioners "burn your (traditional) textbooks" (p. 30).[12] Although this approach may seem radical, it does bring to light the limitations of textbooks for providing information on the cause, diagnosis, prognosis, or treatment of a disorder. To stay up to date in clinical practice, a textbook may need to be revised on a yearly basis.[12] However, research and publication of results in a journal is a deliberative process that often takes years from the germination of an idea, to obtaining funding, carrying out the study, analyzing data, writing up results, submitting to a journal, and waiting out the peer-review process and publication lag for a journal.

The number of scientific publications has increased dramatically since the 1940s.[13] There are an estimated 25,000 scientific journals in the world.[14] Along with this, there are an estimated two million new research papers published each year in the health sciences literature <http://ebm.bmjjournals.com/>. To assimilate the large body of evidence, the practitioner needs to find ways to take advantage of the vast amount of scientific information available, and to find information quickly.

Methods for searching the literature have changed dramatically. Even ten years ago, a practitioner wishing to find information on a particular topic would speak with a librarian and inform him or her of the type of information being sought, perhaps provide a sample article, and help in selecting some key words. The librarian would run the search which would often have to be rerun, depending on whether it captured the desired types of articles. This whole process could take weeks. Given the availability of desktop computer searching, it is now possible for practitioners to conduct their own searches. This allows titles and abstracts to be scanned, provides better information about which articles to copy and read, and makes it possible for the search of electronic databases to be run at any time of the day.

UNDERTAKING A SEARCH OF THE SCIENTIFIC LITERATURE

Although any search algorithm is imperfect, a systematic approach to literature searching can increase the chances of finding pertinent information. Figure 6–1 describes a process for searching the literature and organizing the findings of a search. The following topics provide a step-by-step breakdown of this process.

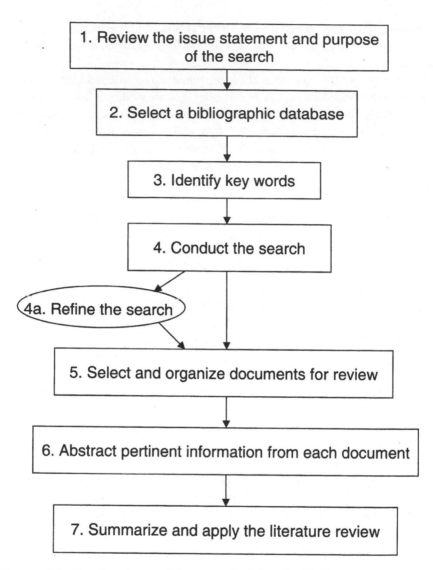

FIGURE 6–1. Flowchart for organizing a search of the scientific literature.

(The later stages [especially steps 5 and 6] of the process are based largely on the Matrix Method, developed by Garrard.)[13] We focus mainly on the use of MEDLINE because it is the largest and most widely available bibliographic database. We also focus on the search for peer-reviewed evidence programs, studies, and data that have been reviewed by other researchers and practitioners.

Review the Issue Statement and Purpose of the Search

Based on the issue statement described in Chapter 4, the purpose of the search should be well outlined. Keep in mind that searching is an iterative process, and a key is the ability to ask one or more answerable questions.[12] While the goal of a search is to identify all relevant material and nothing else, in practice, this is difficult to achieve.[6] The overarching questions include: "Which evidence is relevant to my questions?" and "What conclusions can be drawn regarding effective intervention approaches based on the literature assembled?"[15]

Select a Bibliographic Database

There are numerous bibliographic databases that are now available on-line (Table 6–1). We recommend that readers become familiar with one or more of them. Some of the databases in Table 6–1 require a fee, but if an individual has access to a library, a global fee may already cover the cost. MEDLINE is the most widely used database for searching the biomedical literature. It is maintained by the National Library of Medicine and has several advantages over other databases—it is free to users, updated frequently, and relatively user friendly. MEDLINE does not provide the full text of articles, but rather lists the title, authors, source of the publication, the authors' abstract (if one is available), key word subject headings, and a number of other "tags" that provide information about each publication (Table 6-2).[6] For some journals (e.g., the British Medical Journal), the full text of articles can be linked in, following a MEDLINE search. Numerous other evidence databases exist for a variety of health care specialties and subspecialties.[12] Similar subspecialty databases do not currently exist for public health, so it is recommended that practitioners become familiar with MEDLINE and similar databases in Table 6–1.

Identify Key Words

Key words are terms that describe the characteristics of the subject being reviewed. A useful search strategy is dependent on the sensitivity and precision of the key words used. "Sensitivity" is the ability to identify all relevant material, and "precision" is the amount of relevant material among the information retrieved by the search.[6, 16] Most bibliographic databases require the use of standardized key words. These key words are often found in the list of Medical Subject Heading (MeSH) terms. For a literature search in MEDLINE, these sources of key words are useful (Box 6–1):

Box 6–1. Searching for Evidence on the Effectiveness of Cardiovascular Health Programs

The state "healthy heart" coordinator within the Mississippi Department of Health is in charge of starting a new program in community-based intervention to promote cardiovascular health. She has completed an initial statement of the issue under consideration and now wishes to search the literature. She connects with PubMed via the Internet and begins a search. First, she uses nonstandardized key words, including "cardiovascular disease" and "community intervention." The first run of a search yields 650 citations. Next, she limits the search to literature published in the past ten years; using the same key words, this results in 429 citations. In the third iteration, the same key words are used, literature is limited to the past ten years, and only review articles are selected. This results in 69 citations for which abstracts can be scanned. After scanning these abstracts, the program coordinator obtains copies of the most essential articles.

The coordinator next conducted a second round of searching on the same topic using the standard MeSH terms "Cardiovascular Diseases" and "Health Education." The initial search using these words yielded 4,759 citations, the next search was limited to the past ten years, resulting in 2,177 articles. Finally, the procedure, limited to review articles, yielded 465 citations. This second round of searching resulted in more articles on individual and clinical interventions with a health education component. In this example, the use of nonstandardized key words appeared to better identify the types of articles needed by the coordinator.

---

1. Identify two scientific papers that cover the topic of interest—one more recent and one less recent.[6] These papers can be pulled up on PubMed. In the MEDLINE abstract, a list of MeSH terms will be provided. These can, in turn, be used in subsequent searches.
2. Key words can be found within the alphabetical list of MeSH terms, available on-line at <http://www.nlm.nih.gov/mesh/meshhome.html>.
3. MEDLINE and Current Contents do not require users to use standardized key words. Therefore, you can select your own key words—these are searched for in article titles and abstracts. Generally, using nonstandardized key words provides a less precise literature search than does using standardized terms. However, the MEDLINE interface between standardized and nonstandardized key words allows complete searching without a detailed knowledge of MeSH terms.

Conduct the Search

After the databases and initial key words are identified, it is time to run the search. Once the initial search is run, the number of publications returned will

Table 6–1. Computer-Stored Bibliographic Databases

Database	Dates	Subjects Covered	Fee	Website
MEDLINE® (PubMed)	1966–present	The premier source for bibliographic coverage of biomedical literature; includes references and abstracts from over 4,300 journals	No	\<http://www.nlm.nih.gov/hinfo.html>
Current Contents® (subcategories: Clinical Medicine, Life Sciences, or Social and Behavioral Sciences)	Past year, up-dated weekly	Tables of contents and bibliographic data from current issues of the world's leading scholarly research journals; indexed and loaded within days of publication	Yes	\<http://sunweb.isinet.com/isi/academic/index.html>
PsycINFO®	1887–present	The world's most comprehensive source for bibliographic coverage of psychology and behavioral sciences literature; with special subset files ClinPSYC; databases contain more that 1.5 million records.	Yes	\<http://www.apa.org/psycinfo/>
Dissertation Abstracts Online	1861–present	American and Canadian doctoral dissertations	Yes	\<http://library.dialog.com/bluesheets/html/bl0035.html>
CANCERLIT®	1966–present	Cancer literature from journal articles, government and technical reports, meeting abstracts, special publications, and theses	No	\<http://cancernet.nci.nih.gov/cancerlit.shtml>
TOXLINE®	1980–present	Extensive array of references to literature on biochemical, pharmacological, physiological, and toxicological effects of drugs and other chemicals.	No	\<http://toxnet.nlm.nih.gov/index.html>

Table 6–2. Selected Tags Used to Index Articles in MEDLINE

Category	Subcategory
Publication type	Clinical trial
	Editorial
	Letter
	Meta-analysis
	Practice guideline
	Randomized controlled trial
	Review
Gender	Female
	Male
Language	English
	French
	German
	Italian
	Japanese
	Russian
	Spanish
Publication date	YYYY/MM/DD (month and day are optional)

Source: Adapted from Petitti.[6]

likely be large and include many irrelevant articles. Several features of MED-LINE (PubMed) can assist searchers in limiting the scope of the search to the most relevant articles. Figure 6–2 shows a partial listing from a PubMed search using the key words "evidence-based public health."

- Specific designations such as "editorial," "letter," or "comment" can be excluded. Searches can also be limited to English-language publications, to a certain date of publication, or to a gender (Table 6–2). These tags are found by clicking the "Limits" icon.
- An initial search can focus on review articles by selecting the publication type. This allows a search of the citation list of review articles in order to identify original research articles of particular interest.
- PubMed will allow you to link to other "related articles" by simply clicking an icon on the right side of each citation.
- If a particularly useful article is found, the author's name can be searched for other similar studies. The same author will often have multiple publications on the same subject. To avoid irrelevant retrievals, you should use the author's last name and first and middle initials in the search.
- In nearly every case, it is necessary to refine the search approach. As articles are identified, the key word and search strategy will be refined and improved through a "snowballing" technique that allows users to gain familiarity with

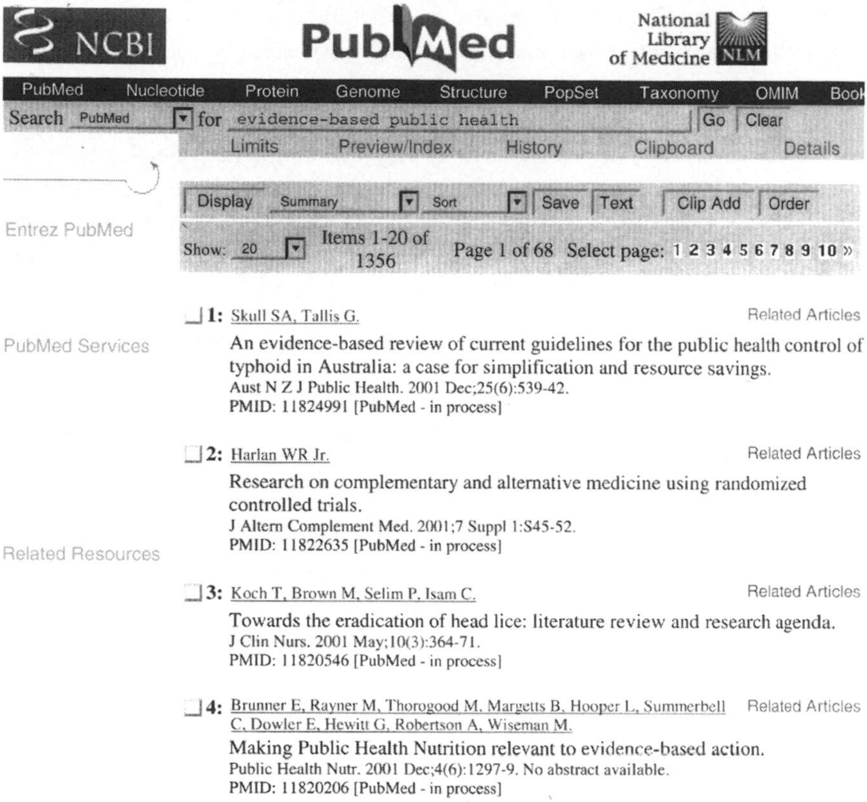

FIGURE 6–2. Web page for a PubMed literature search <http://www.nlm.nih.gov>.

the literature and gather more useful articles.[13] Articles that may be useful can be saved during each session by clicking "Add to Clipboard" within PubMed.

Select and Organize Documents for Review

Once a set of articles has been located, it is time to organize the documents.[13] This will set the stage for abstracting the pertinent information. Generally, it is helpful to organize the documents by the type of study (original research, review article, review article with quantitative synthesis, guideline, etc.). It is often useful to enter documents into a reference management database such as EndNote® <http://www.endnote.com> or ProCite® <http://www.procite. com>. These software applications allow users to switch from one reference format to another when producing reports and grant applications and to download journal citations directly from the World Wide Web, eliminating the chance for typing errors. These packages also have helpful search and sort capabilities. A systematic method of organizing the articles themselves is essential. A limited number of articles on a certain topic can be kept in a three-ring binder, but larger bodies of evidence may be entered in a reference management database such as EndNote® by key word; articles can then be filed alphabetically by the last name of the first author of each article or simply with an identification number. This allows users to search a database by key word later in the research process.

Abstract Pertinent Information from Each Document

When a group of articles has been assembled, the next step is to create an evidence matrix—a spreadsheet with rows and columns that allows users to abstract the key information from each article.[13] Creating a matrix provides a structure for putting the information in order. In developing a matrix, the choice of column topics is a key consideration. It is often useful to consider both methodologic characteristics and content-specific results as column headings. A sample review matrix is shown in Table 6–3. In this example, studies were also organized within rows by an ecological framework, described in detail in Chapter 8. As you get more experienced at searching the literature and organizing results, you may wish to modify column headings slightly.

Summarize and Apply the Literature Review

Once a body of studies has been abstracted into a matrix, the literature may be summarized for various purposes. For example, you many need to provide background information for a new budget item that is being presented to the administrator of an agency. Knowing the best intervention science should increase the chances of convincing key policy makers of the need for a particular program or policy. You may also need to summarize the literature in order to build the case for a grant application that seeks external support for a particular program.

SEEKING SOURCES OUTSIDE THE SEARCHABLE LITERATURE

A great deal of important evidence on public health topics is not found in published journal articles and books.[6, 17] Reasons for the limitations of searching the published literature include the following: (1) many researchers and practitioners fail to write up their research because of competing projects and other time demands; (2) journal editors are faced with difficult decisions on what to publish and there may be a tendency toward publishing "positive" studies (publication bias), and (3) in some areas of the world, lack of resources precludes systematic empirical research.[18] The following approaches should prove useful in finding evidence beyond the scientific literature.

The "Fugitive" Literature

The "fugitive" or "grey" literature includes government reports, book chapters, conference proceedings, and other materials that are not found in on-line databases such as MEDLINE.[6, 19] These are particularly important in attempting a summary of the literature involving meta-analysis or cost-effectiveness analysis (see Chapter 3). It can be difficult to locate the fugitive literature. Experts on the topic of interest are probably the best source of information—you can write or e-mail key informants asking them to provide information on relevant published literature that would not be identified through database searching. More broad-based searches can be conducted of the World Wide Web using search engines such as Dogpile <http://www.dogpile.com>, Google <http://www.google.com>, or MetaCrawler <http://www.metacrawler.com>. The advantage of these searches is their ability to find a large number of sources. The main disadvantage is the user's lack of control over the quality of the information returned. Information collected from a wide search of the Web must be viewed with a critical eye.[20] The CRISP (Computer Retrieval of Information on Scientific Projects) database, maintained by the U.S. National Institutes of Health provides summaries of funded research projects that can be useful in finding information prior to its appearance in the peer-reviewed literature <http://www-commons.cit.nih.gov/crisp/>.

Key Informant Interviews

Often a public health practitioner wants to understand not only the outcomes of a program or policy but also the process of developing and carrying out an intervention (see Chapter 9). Many process issues are difficult to glean from the scientific literature because the methods sections in published articles may not be comprehensive enough to show all aspects of the intervention. A program may evolve over time and what is in the published literature may differ from what is currently being done. In addition, many good program and policy evaluations go unpublished.

In these cases, key informant interviews may be useful. Key informants are experts on a certain topic and may include a university researcher who has years of experience in a particular intervention area or a local program manager who

Table 6–3. Example Evidence Matrix for Literature on Physical Activity Promotion at Various Levels of an Ecological Framework

Lead Author, Article Title, Journal Citation	Year	Study Design	METHODOLOGIC CHARACTERISTICS				CONTENT-SPECIFIC FINDINGS		
			Study Population	Sample Size	Intervention Characteristics	Results	Conclusions	Other Comments
Individual Level								
Brownson et al. Patterns and correlates of physical activity among women aged 40 years and older, United States. *American Journal Public Health* 2000; 90:264–270	2000	Cross-sectional	Ethnically diverse U.S. women, aged 40 yrs. and older	2,912	N/A—not an intervention	Physical activity lowest among African American & American Indian women (odds ratios = 1.35 and 1.65); 72% of women were active based on a composite definition. Rural women were less active than urban dwellers	Minority women are among the least active subgroups in America	Cross-sectional nature limits causal inferences; Telephone survey data may not be entirely representative
Interpersonal Level								
Simons et al. A pilot urban church-based program to reduce risk factors for diabetes among Western Samoans in New Zealand. *Diabetic Medicine* 1998;15:136–142	1998	Prospective; non-randomized	Western Samoan church members, South Auckland, New Zealand; 34% male, 66% female	Intervention = 78; control = 144	Social support, health education, supervised & structured exercise	Weight remained stable in the intervention church but increased in the control church (p = 0.05). In the intervention church, there was an associated reduction in waist circumference, p <0.001), an increase in diabetes knowledge, p <0.001) and an increase in the proportion exercising regularly, p <0.05).	Diabetes risk reduction programs based upon lifestyle change, diabetes awareness, and empowerment of high risk communities can significantly reduce risk factors for future Type 2 diabetes	Participation rates: Introductory talk = 93%; Video session = 18%; Exercise session = 84%

Organizational Level

Citation	Year	Design	N	Population	Intervention	Results	Conclusion	Comments
Sharpe et al. Exercise beliefs and behaviors among older employees: a health promotion trial. *Gerontologist* 1992;32:444–449.	1992	Group randomized by worksite unit	250 initially, 121 used for analysis	University employees, ages 50–69, 53% male, 91% White, 6% Black	Health counseling and exercise	The change in walking or other exercise from baseline to 1-year follow-up was not significantly different between intervention and control groups.	Baseline exercise frequency was the only predictor of exercise behavior 1 year later.	

Community Level

Citation	Year	Design	N	Population	Intervention	Results	Conclusion	Comments
King et al. Increasing exercise among blue-collar employees: the tailoring of worksite programs to meet specific needs. *Preventive Medicine* 1988;17(3): 357–65.	1988	Prospective; quasi-experimental	22	Employees at Stanford University skilled trade division, Palo Alto, CA; 100% men; mean age, 45 yrs	-week exercise program using an on-site par-course, and incorporating such motivational strategies as public monitoring, inter-shop competition, and activity-based incentives	Participants showed increases in fitness levels ($p < 0.0001$) & decreases in weight ($p < 0.05$) compared with nonparticipants; Attendees also showed greater confidence about the ability to exercise	Low cost program appears to influence fitness and weight	Long-term program adherence needs to be studied

Health Policy Level

Citation	Year	Design	N	Population	Intervention	Results	Conclusion	Comments
Linenger et al. Physical fitness gains following simple environmental change. *America Journal Preventive Medicine* 1991 7(5):298–310	1991	Non-randomized group trial	2,372	San Diego naval air station community members (intervention) and 2 control communities; 85% male in intervention site	Modification of physical environment (e.g., bike paths, new equipment, athletic events); Organizational policy intervention (release time encouraged)	Significant improvement in physical readiness test (PRT) and 1.5 mi. run in intervention community compared with either control community or a Navy-wide sample; 12.4% failed the PRT in 1987 compared with 5.1% in 1988 in the intervention site	A relatively simple program improved fitness performance	The generalizability to a nonmilitary population should be considered

has the field experience to know what works when it comes to designing and implementing effective interventions. There are several steps in carrying out a "key informant" process:

1. Identify the key informants who might be useful for gathering information. They can be found in the literature, via professional networks, and increasingly, on the Internet <see http://www.profnet.com>.
2. Determine the types of information needed. It is often helpful to write out a short list of open-ended questions that are of particular interest. This can help in framing a conversation and making the most efficient use of time. Prior to a conversation with an expert, it is useful to e-mail him or her your questions so they begin thinking about replies.
3. Collect the data. This often can be accomplished via a 15 to 20 minute phone conversation if the questions of interest are well framed ahead of time.
4. Summarize the data collected. Conversations can be recorded and transcribed using formative research techniques. More often, good notes are taken and conversations recorded to end up with a series of bullet points from each key informant conversation.
5. Conduct follow-up, as needed. As with literature searching, key informant interviews often result in a snowballing effect in which one expert identifies another who is also knowledgeable. As information becomes repetitious, the data collector can decide when enough information has been collected.

Professional Meetings

Annually, there are dozens of relevant and helpful professional meetings in public health, ranging from large conventions such as that of the American Public Health Association to smaller, specialty meetings such as the annual meeting on diabetes prevention and control. Important intervention research is often presented at these meetings. The smaller venues allow one to talk informally with the researcher to learn details of his or her work and how it might apply in a particular setting. Practitioners should seek out meetings that use a peer-review process for abstract review, helping to ensure that high quality research is presented. Meetings generally provide a list of presenters and abstracts of presentations prior to or during the meeting. The main limitation for many practitioners is the inability to attend a variety of professional meetings because of limited travel funds.

SUMMARY

Literature searching can be an inexact science because of the wide scope of public health and inconsistencies in search strategies.[21] But a systematic search of the literature is key for evidence-based decision making.

Essential points in this chapter include the following:

- It is important to understand the various uses of different types professional literature i.e., original research articles, review articles, reviews with quantitative synthesis, and guidelines.
- A step-by-step approach to literature searching will improve the sensitivity and precision of the process.
- Other valuable sources of scientific information can include the fugitive literature, key informant interviews, and professional meetings.
- Although this chapter attempts to provide the essential information for locating scientific information quickly, there is no substitute for trying out these approaches and customizing procedures to your own needs.

SUGGESTED READINGS AND WEBSITES

Readings

Garrard J. *Health Sciences Literature Review Made Easy. The Matrix Method.* Gaithersburg, MD: Aspen Publishers, Inc., 1999.
Greenhalgh T. How to read a paper. Getting your bearings (deciding what the paper is about). *British Medical Journal* 1997;315:243–246.

Selected Websites

The Agency for Healthcare Research and Quality <http://www.ahrq.gov/>. The Agency for Healthcare Research and Quality (AHRQ) research provides evidence-based information on health care outcomes, quality, and cost, use, and access. Information from AHRQ's research helps people make more informed decisions and improve the quality of health care services. AHRQ was formerly known as the Agency for Health Care Policy and Research.

Annual Review of Public Health <http://publhealth.annualreviews.org/>. The mission of Annual Reviews is to provide systematic, periodic examinations of scholarly advances in a number of scientific fields through critical authoritative reviews. The comprehensive critical review not only summarizes a topic but also roots out errors of fact or concept and provokes discussion that will lead to new research activity. The critical review is an essential part of the scientific method.

National Academy of Sciences: Institute of Medicine <http://www.iom.edu/>. The mission of the Institute of Medicine is to advance and disseminate scientific knowledge to improve human health. The Institute provides objective, timely, authoritative information and advice concerning health and science policy to government, the corporate sector, the professions and the public.

Partners in Information Access for Public Health Professionals <http://nnlm.gov/partners/>. A collaborative project to provide public health professionals with timely, convenient access to information resources to help them improve the health of the American public.

REFERENCES

1. Jones R, Kinmonth A-L. *Critical Reading for Primary Care*. Oxford: Oxford University Press, 1995.
2. Greenhalgh T. How to read a paper. Getting your bearings (deciding what the paper is about). *British Medical Journal* 1997;315:243–246.
3. The Annual Review of Public Health. Available at: <www.AnnualReviews.org, 2001>.
4. Breslow RA, Ross SA, Weed DL. Quality of reviews in epidemiology. *American Journal of Public Health* 1998;88(3):475–477.
5. Glass GV. Primary, secondary and meta-analysis of research. *Educational Research* 1976;5:3–8.
6. Petitti DB. *Meta-analysis, Decision Analysis, and Cost-Effectiveness Analysis: Methods for Quantitative Synthesis in Medicine*. 2nd ed. New York: Oxford University Press, 2000.
7. Canadian Task Force on the Periodic Health Examination. The periodic health examination. *Canadian Medical Association Journal* 1979;121:1193–1254.
8. Truman BI, Smith-Akin CK, Hinman AR, al e. Developing the guide to community preventive services—overview and rationale. *American Journal of Preventive Medicine* 2000;18(1S):18–26.
9. U.S. Preventive Services Task Force. *Guide to Clinical Preventive Services*. 2nd ed. Baltimore: Williams & Wilkins, 1996.
10. Woolf SH, DiGuiseppi CG, Atkins D, Kamerow DB. Developing evidence-based clinical practice guidelines: Lessons learned by the U.S. Preventive Services Task Force. *Annual Review of Public Health* 1996;17:511–538.
11. Last JM, ed. *A Dictionary of Epidemiology*. 4th ed. New York: Oxford University Press, 2001.
12. Sackett DL, Straus SE, Richardson WS, Rosenberg W, Haynes RB. *Evidence-Based Medicine. How to Practice and Teach EBM*. 2nd ed. Edinburgh: Churchill Livingston, 2000.
13. Garrard J. *Health Sciences Literature Review Made Easy. The Matrix Method*. Gaithersburg, MD: Aspen Publishers, Inc., 1999.
14. Johnson T. Shattuck lecture: Medicine and the media. *New England Journal of Medicine* 1998;339:87–92.
15. Bartholomew LK, Parcel GS, Kok G, Gottlieb NH. *Intervention Mapping. Designing Theory- and Evidence-Based Health Promotion Programs*. Mountain View, CA: Mayfield Publishing Company, 2001.

16. Dickersin K, Scherer R, Lefebvre C. Identifying relevant studies for systematic reviews. *British Medical Journal* 1994;309(6964):1286–1291.
17. Muir Gray JA. *Evidence-Based Healthcare: How to Make Health Policy and Management Decisions*. New York and Edinburgh: Churchill Livingstone, 1997.
18. McQueen D. Strengthing the evidence base for health promotion. Paper presented at the Fifth Global Conference for Health Promotion. Health Promotion: Bridging the Equity Gap Mexico City, June 5–9, 2000.
19. Hart C. *Doing a Literature Search. A Comprehensive Guide for the Social Sciences*. Thousand Oaks, CA: Sage Publications Inc., 2001.
20. Schindler JV, Middleton C. Conducting public health research on the World Wide Web. *The International Electronic Journal of Health Education* 2001;4:308–317.
21. Rimer BK, Glanz DK, Rasband G. Searching for evidence about health education and health behavior interventions. *Health Education and Health Behavior* 2001; 28(2):231–248.

7

Developing and Prioritizing Program Options

A decision is as good as the information that goes into it.
—John F. Bookout, Jr.

When one is implementing an evidence-based process, numerous program and policy options become apparent. Identifying and choosing among these options are not simple, straightforward tasks. The preceding chapters were designed to help readers define a problem and develop a broad array of choices. For example, methods from descriptive epidemiology and public health surveillance can be used to characterize the magnitude of a particular issue and tools such as economic evaluation are useful in assessing the benefits of an intervention compared with the costs.

After options are identified, priorities need to be set among various alternatives. In general, methods for setting priorities are better developed for clinical interventions than for community approaches, in part because there is a larger body of evidence on the effectiveness of clinical interventions than on that of community-based studies. There is also a larger base of cost-effectiveness studies of clinical interventions. However, it is unlikely that even the most conscientious and well-intentioned clinician will incorporate all recommended preventive services during each visit by a patient, given competing demands.[1,2] In community settings many of the tools and approaches for identifying and prioritizing interventions are still being developed and tested.

This chapter is divided into four main sections. The first describes some broad-based considerations to take into account when examining options and priorities. The next section outlines analytic methods and models that have been applied when setting clinical and community priorities in health promotion and disease prevention. The third section is an overview of the concepts of innovation and creativity in option selection. And the final section describes the development and uses of analytic frameworks in developing and prioritizing options.

BACKGROUND

Resources are always limited in public health; in many ways programs in public health represent a "zero-sum game." That is, the total available resources for public health programs and services are not likely to increase substantially from year to year. Only rarely are there exceptions to this scenario, such as the multibillion dollar settlements of tobacco lawsuits that, in some areas of the United States, are resulting in substantial public health spending and benefits.[3] Therefore, careful, evidence-based examination of program options is necessary to ensure that the most effective approaches to improving the public's health are taken. The key is to follow a process that is both systematic and objective, combining science with the realities of the environment.[4]

At a macrolevel, part of the goal in setting priorities carefully is to shift from resource-based decision-making to a population-based process. To varying degrees this occurred in the United States during the twentieth century. In the resource-based planning cycle, the spiral of increased resources and increased demand for resources helped to drive the cost of health care services continually higher, even as the health status of some population groups declined.[5] In contrast, the population-based planning cycle gives greater attention to population needs and outcomes, including quality of life, and has been described as the starting point in decision making.[5] This approach is the desired framework now and is either implicitly or explicitly followed throughout this chapter.

When one is examining options, there are at least six different sources of information, including several that have been discussed in earlier chapters. These sources can be grouped in two broad categories: scientific information and "other expert" information. Among scientific sources, the practitioner might seek program options derived from peer-reviewed sources; this might include journal articles or evidence-based summary documents such as clinical or community guidelines. Within the broad group of "other expert" information, one might seek input from professional colleagues in the workplace, at professional meetings, or via key stakeholders (see Chapter 4). Overarching all of these categories is the mechanism for identifying options. Electronic mechanisms such as the Internet can be especially promising in this regard for busy practitioners. Using the Internet, program options can be rapidly scanned from a desktop computer. Some excellent examples of useful Internet sites are provided at the end of this chapter.

As options are being considered and a course of action determined, it is important to distinguish decision making from problem solving. Problem solving involves the determination of one correct solution; it is like solving a mathematical problem. In contrast, decision making in organizations is the process of making a choice from among a set of rational alternatives. In choosing a public health approach, there is often not one "correct" answer but rather a set of options to be identified and prioritized. Most significant decision making in public health organizations occurs in the context of uncertainty. Epidemiologic uncertainty in study design and interpretation was discussed in Chapters 2 and 5. Other influences on the decision-making process include politics, legal issues, economic forces, and societal values. Modern decision-making theory also recognizes that individual decision makers are influenced by their values, unconscious reflexes, skills, and habits.[6] Key elements for effective decision making in the context of uncertainty include

• Acquiring sufficient evidence on all alternatives
• Approaching the problem in a rational and systematic fashion
• Relying on experience, intuition, and judgment

It is also important to understand that decision making often involves some element of risk and that these risks can occur at various levels. At the program level, the program option chosen may not be the optimal choice or may not be implemented properly, thus limiting the ability to reach objectives. Within an organization, program staff may be hesitant to provide objective data on various options, especially when a negative outcome could lead to program discontinuation (and loss of jobs). But an organization and leaders who support creativity and innovation will encourage new ideas even when risk is present.

ANALYTIC METHODS FOR PRIORITIZING HEALTH ISSUES AND PROGRAM OPTIONS

There are many different ways of prioritizing program and policy issues in public health practice. Although it is unlikely that "one size fits all," several tools and resources have proven useful for practitioners in a variety of settings.[7] In addition to using various analytic methods, priority setting will occur at different geographic and political levels. An entire country may establish broad health priorities. In the Netherlands, a comprehensive approach was applied to health services delivery that included an investment in health technology assessment, use of guidelines, and development of criteria to determine priority on waiting lists. Underlying this approach was the belief that excluding certain

---

Box 7–1. Prioritizing Environmental Interventions to Prevent Obesity

Obesity is increasing at such a rate that some now consider it a pandemic. Researchers from New Zealand and Australia proposed an ecological framework for understanding obesity that included influences of biology, individual behavior, and the environment.[12] With this framework, they developed the ANGELO model that has been used to prioritize the settings and sectors for interventions to address obesity. The ANGELO method utilizes a grid that includes two sizes of environments on one axis (i.e., microsettings, such as neighborhoods and schools, and macrosectors such as transportation systems and health care systems). On the other axis, four types of environments (physical, economic, political, and sociocultural) are mapped. This framework has been pilot-tested in Torres Islands, Australia, where data were collected from group and individual (stakeholder) interviews among local residents and health workers. Stakeholders generated a long list of potential "obesogenic" elements and ranked each according to the perceived relevance to their community and their potential changeability. In its initial applications, the ANGELO framework has proven useful in stimulating brainstorming among stakeholders and prioritizing future topics for intervention and research.[12]

---

health care services was necessary to ensure access of all citizens to essential health care.[8] In other instances, an individual state or province may conduct a priority-setting process. Based on the recommendations of an eleven-member group of consumers and health care professionals, the state of Oregon ranked public health services covered under its Medicaid program, using cost-effectiveness analysis and various qualitative measures, to extend coverage for high priority services to a greater number of the state's poor residents.[9, 10] These approaches often need to take community values into account. In Oregon, for example, a series of forty-seven community meetings resulted in a grouping of thirteen key values into three categories: value to society, value to an individual in need of a service, and attributes that are essential to basic health care (e.g., prevention, quality of life).[8, 11] Experience in New Zealand and Australia shows that stakeholder input can be valuable in priority setting (Box 7–1).[12]

Many of the same approaches that have been applied at a macrolevel can be used to prioritize programs or policies within a public health or voluntary health agency, within a health care organization, or at a city or county level.

Prioritizing Clinical Issues and Interventions

There have been few systematic attempts to develop and apply objective criteria for prioritizing clinical preventive services. As noted in Chapter 3, prioritization of clinical interventions tends to benefit from the development of guidelines for

Table 7–1. Priorities among Recommended Clinical Preventive Services[a]

Services	CPB	CE	Total
Vaccinate children: *DTP/DTaP, MMR, Oral Polio/IPV, Hib, Hep B, Varicella*	5	5	10
Assess adults for tobacco use and provide tobacco cessation counseling	5	4	9
Screen for vision impairment among adults 65+ years	4	5	9
Assess adolescents for drinking and drug use and counsel on alcohol and drug abstinence	3	5	8[b,c]
Assess adolescents for tobacco use and provide an anti-tobacco message or advice to quit	4	4	8[b]
Screen for cervical cancer among sexually active women or 18+ years	5	3	8
Screen for colorectal cancer (FOBT and/or sigmoidoscopy) among all persons 50+ years	5	3	8
Screen for hemoglobinopathies, PKU, and congenital hypothyroidism among newborns	3	5	8
Screen for hypertension among all persons	5	3	8
Vaccinate adults 65+ years against influenza	4	4	8
Screen for chlamydia among women 15–24 years	3	4	7[b]
Screen for high blood cholesterol among men 35–65 years and women 45–65 years	5	2	7
Screen for problem drinking among adults and provide brief counseling	4	3	7[b]
Vaccinate adults 65+ years against pneumococcal disease	2	5	7
Assess infant feeding practices and provide counseling on:	1	5	6
Breastfeeding; use of iron-enriched foods; risk of baby bottle tooth decay			
Assess risk of STDs (including HIV) and provide counseling on measures to reduce risk	3	3	6[b]
Screen for breast cancer (mammography alone or with CBE) among women ages 50–69 years	4	2	6
Screen for vision impairment at age 3–4 years	2	4	6[b]
Assess oral health practices and provide counseling on:	3	2	5[b]
Brushing and flossing daily; visiting a dental care provider regularly			

(Continued)

primary care providers. These include the efforts of the Canadian Task Force on the Periodic Health Examination[13] and the U.S. Preventive Services Task Force.[14]

One approach to prioritizing clinical preventive services was recently proposed by Coffield and colleagues.[15, 16] This approach is being developed in conjunction with the publication of the third edition of the *Guide to Clinical Preventive Services*. With analytic methods, clinical interventions were ranked according to two dimensions: burden of disease prevented by each service and average cost-effectiveness. Burden was described by the clinically preventable burden (CPB): the amount of disease that would be prevented by a particular service in usual practice if the service were delivered to 100% of the target population. CPB was measured in quality-adjusted life years (QALYs), as defined in Chapter 3. Cost-effectiveness (CE) was the ratio of net costs to burden of disease prevented i.e., (costs of prevention–costs averted) / QALYs saved.

Table 7–1. (*Continued*)

Services	CPB	CE	Total
Assess the safety practices of parents of children 0–4 years and provide counseling on: *Child safety seats; window/stair guards; pool fence; poison control; hot water temp; bicycle helmet*	1	4	5[b]
Counsel on risks/benefits of hormone replacement among peri- and postmenopausal women	4	1	5[b]
Assess calcium/vitamin D intake of adolescent and adult women and counsel on use of supplements	2	2	4[b]
Assess folic acid intake among women of childbearing age and counsel on use of supplements	1	3	4[b]
Assess physical activity patterns of all persons over age 2 and counsel on increasing activity levels	3	1	4[b]
Provide newborns with ocular prophylaxis to protect against gonococcal eye disease	1	3	4[b]
Screen for hearing impairment among persons 65+ years	2	2	4[b]
Assess dietary patterns of persons over age 2 and provide counseling on: *Intake of fat/cholesterol; caloric balance; intake of fruits, vegetables, grains*	2	1	3
Assess the safety practices of all persons over age 4 and provide counseling on: *Seat belt use; smoke detector use; firearm storage/removal from home; bicycle/ motorcycle helmet use; dangers of alcohol use; protection against slip and fall hazards for older persons*	2	1	3[b]
Screen for rubella among women of childbearing age using serology and/or history and vaccinate	1	1	2
Vaccinate all persons against tetanus-diphtheria (Td boosters)	1	1	2

[a]Services are those recommended by the U.S. Preventive Services Task Force for average risk patients in the *Guide to Clinical Preventive Services, 2nd edition.*

[b]Services for which total scores have greater uncertainty. See Maciosek et al.[16] for explanation.

[c]Services in **bold type** are those with scores of 7+ for which available data indicate that delivery to the U.S. population eligible for the services is less than or equal to 50%.

Each service was assigned CPB and CE scores from 1 to 5 (according to quintile), with 5 being the best possible score. The rankings were added so that each service ended up with a final score from 2 to 10 (Table 7–1). It is worth noting that scores are not proportionate, e.g., a total score of 8 is more valuable but not necessarily twice as valuable as a total score of 4.[16] With this method, the two interventions with the highest priority rankings were counseling for tobacco cessation and vaccination of children to prevent a variety of infectious diseases.

There have also been attempts to develop and apply criteria for prioritizing health behaviors for populations, using the epidemiologic concept of risk and, in some cases, applying it to economic costs. One such model is the Health Risk Appraisal (HRA). HRA evolved from a counseling tool that physicians and health educators used with their patients into a simulation model that projects results of behavior change programs targeted at particular populations. The HRA contains three essential features: (1) an assessment of personal health habits and risk factors based on questionnaire responses from the patient or client; (2) a quantitative or qualitative assessment of an individual's future risk of death or adverse health outcomes; and (3) the provision of educational messages on ways of reducing health risks.[17] Outcome results can be assessed as savings attributed to medical costs for numerous health behaviors.[18]

Prioritizing Public Health Issues at the Community Level

There are both qualitative and quantitative approaches to setting public health priorities for communities. Although many and diverse definitions of "community have been offered," we define it as a group of individuals that shares attributes of place, social interaction, and social and political responsibility.[19] In practice, many data systems are organized geographically and therefore communities are often defined by place. A sound priority-setting process can help generate widespread support for public health issues when it is well documented and endorsed by communities.[7]

Multiple groups of researchers and practitioners have proposed standardized criteria for prioritizing public health issues at the community level.[4, 7, 20–24] Each of these methods differs, but they have at least three common elements. First, each relies on some measure of burden, whether measured in mortality, morbidity, or years of potential life lost. Each method also attempts to quantify preventability (i.e., the potential effects of intervention). And finally, resource issues are often addressed in the decision making process, both in terms of costs of intervention and of the resources of an organization to carry out a particular program or policy. Two analytical methods frequently used as auxiliary in the prioritization process are economic appraisal and an approach based on comparison with "ideal" or "achievable" population health status.[25] Several approaches to categorizing and prioritizing various interventions that use the three common elements will be discussed briefly here as well as one example each of the approaches based on economic data and achievable population health status.

A relatively straightforward way of categorizing program and policy options has been presented by Green and Kreuter (Table 7–2).[26] Within this 2 × 2 framework, options can be categorized according to their importance and changeability. Importance might be based on burden of disease, injury, impairment, or exposure. Changeability is synonymous with preventability. Within this framework, options in the upper left and lower right cells are relatively easy to prioritize. Those in the lower left and upper right are more difficult to assess. A highly important issue but one about which little is known from a preventive standpoint should be the focus of innovation in program development. A strong

Table 7–2. Considerations in Setting Program Priorities

	More Important	*Less Important*
More changeable	Highest priority for program focus	Low priority except to demonstrate change for political or other purpose
	Example: interventions to improve vaccination coverage in children, adolescents, and adults	*Example*: programs to prevent work-related pneumoconiosis
Less changeable	Priority for innovative program with evaluation essential	No intervention program
	Example: programs to prevent mental impairment and disability	*Example*: policies to improve emergency response to natural disasters

Source: adapted from Green and Kreuter.[26]

focus on evaluation should be maintained in this category so that new programs can be assessed for effectiveness. A program or policy in the upper right corner might be initiated for political, social, or cultural reasons.

Using a different process, the Maryland Department of Health in cooperation with twenty-four local jurisdictions has established a prioritization process based on consensus indicators and comparisons with U.S. rates and trends (Figure 7–1).[7] They refer to their model as the "golden diamond." It permits state and local comparisons of various endpoints, based on morbidity and mortality rates. Ranks are used to help decide where state and local resources should be focused. This initial prioritization is based solely on data and does not include qualitative factors. One of its major advantages is that it is based on existing data sets and is therefore relatively easy to carry out.

A third approach to prioritization, largely based on quantitative methods, was proposed by Hanlon and Pickett[21] and further elaborated by Vilnius and Dandoy.[4] The model, the Basic Priority Rating (BPR), is based on the following formula:

$$BPR = [(A + B) C] / 3 \times D$$

where A is the size of the problem, B the seriousness of the problem, C the effectiveness of intervention, and D is propriety, economics, acceptability, resources, and legality (known as PEARL). Values for each part of the formula are converted from rates and ratings to scores. As an illustration, Table 7–3 provides an application of the BPR formula for a set of public health issues. Assumptions and judgments are required in using this method, since some aspects of the process, such as determination of PEARL, are fairly subjective. Finer details of this method are available in the original publications.[4, 21]

Priority Rank

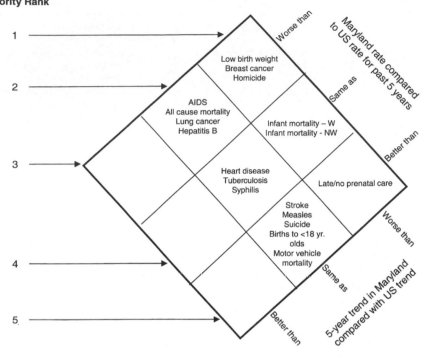

FIGURE 7–1. Consensus set of indicators and priority ranks for Maryland, 1989–1994.

In another example, the Missouri Department of Health and Senior Services applied a simplified two-step method of prioritization to surveillance-derived data.[27] In the first step, statewide disease and health condition indicators were grouped into three sets: magnitude (emergency room visits and hospitalizations), severity (overall mortality and mortality before age 65) and urgency (trend in mortality). Equally weighted indicator categories were used to rank diseases and conditions. For each condition, the rankings of magnitude, severity, and urgency were summed to generate a final overall ranking score. Diseases and conditions were prioritized, based on natural break of the list of ranked scores. This step of the prioritization model also incorporated adhoc literature information on interventions with known effectiveness. In the second step, the county-specific morbidity (combined number of emergency room visits and hospitalizations) and number of deaths for each of the seventeen top priority diseases and conditions identified in the first step were compared with the state average. The differences in either morbidity or mortality between a county and the state were classified as same/lower, higher, and statistically significantly higher, using statistical testing for proportions. For each county, the statistically significant values were tallied across all diseases and conditions to generate a final score. The ranking

Table 7–3. Use of the Basic Priority Rating (BPR) for Four Public Health Issues

	PUBLIC HEALTH ISSUE			
Criteria	HIV/AIDS	Coronary Heart Disease	Motor Vehicle Injuries	Cigarette Smoking
Size				
Incidence/prevalence[a]	26.7	3,058	176	10,000
Incidence/prevalence score	2	6	4	8
Mortality[a]	16.4	280.7	18.0	44.1
Mortality score	2	4	2	2
Overall size score (A = average of incidence/prevalence score and mortality score) (scale of 1–10)	2	5	3	5
Seriousness				
Urgency score[b]	3	1	2	0
Severity				
Case fatality rate	1.0	0.06	0.10	0.004
Case fatality score	5	3	3	1
Years of potential life lost (YPLL)	35.0	13.3	43.7	1.9
YPLL score	5	3	5	0
Average severity score	5	3	4	0.5
Economic loss (case cost/year in $)	50,151	8,700	45,500	643
Economic loss score	5	2	5	1
Impact on others score[b]	5	1	3	2
Overall seriousness score (B = urgency score + average severity score + economic loss score + impact on others score) (scale of 0–20)	18	7	14	3.5
Effectiveness of Intervention				
Program efficacy %	30	50	40	60
Target potential %	30	70	60	90
Overall effectiveness score (C = program efficacy X target potential) (scale of 0–10)	0.9	3.5	2.4	5.4
PEARL (D)[c]	1	1	1	1
Total BPR score =[(A + B) C]/3 X D	6	14	13.6	15.3
Overall ranking	4	2	3	1

Sources: Hanlon and Pickett,[21] Vilnius and Dandoy,[4] Zaza et al.[24]

[a]Rate per 100,000.

[b]Lacks a clearly defined data source; relies on science, knowledge, and public opinion.

[c]Includes propriety, economics, acceptability, resources, and legality.

of this final score, from highest to lowest priority, identified the counties with significantly higher morbidity and mortality than the state, based on the seventeen priority diseases and conditions. This information was displayed in maps to identify each of the priority diseases and conditions and to prioritize by geographical area (county). For each condition, map colors reflected the three possible classifications of mortality and morbidity in each county in relation to the state: significantly higher than state, higher than state, same/less than state. These data are available from the Missouri Department of Health and Senior Services <http://www.dhss.state.mo.us>.

Economic approaches vary from a simple estimate of the cost associated with the attributable risk of a condition (e.g., obesity, alcoholism) to a more complex assessment of the costs, benefits, and effectiveness of interventions. In the former approach, customarily, the population attributable risk (PAR) measure for a condition is used to extrapolate its expected costs to the population as expressed by the disease it affects.[28] Often, one has to accommodate the fact that there are some situations in which many factors affect one disease and that there are others in which one disease is affected by many factors.[29, 30] Because the PAR estimates the amount of disease that could be prevented through reduction of risk factor(s), the PAR for many important and prevalent risk factors have been calculated and published.[31–33] In addition, the economic costs of a given health condition or risk factor can be estimated. For example, Wolff and Colditz estimated the costs associated with obesity in the United States.[28] This type of information can be incorporated in models, such as those proposed by Vilnius and Dandoy,[4] as another summary measure to be scored and ranked. The techniques, examples and limitations of such economic evaluations are described in Chapter 3.

The prioritization approach, based on comparison of a population health problem with the "ideal" or "achievable" population health status, is frequently used to advance the policy decision-making process by singling out an objective, limited set of health problems. It usually involves identifying desirable or achievable levels for an epidemiological measure such as mortality, incidence, or prevalence. One such approach used the lowest achieved mortality rate, calculated from mortality rates that actually have been achieved by some population or population segment at some time and place, and risk-eliminated mortality rates, estimated by mortality levels that would have been achieved with elimination of known-risk factors.[25] A variation of this approach can be used to identify disparities related to race-ethnicity, gender, or other groupings of populations. Similar approaches have been applied in Maine,[34] St. Louis, Missouri,[35] and among all counties of Missouri.[36] Results of such assessments can be incorporated in the previously described models by Hanlon-Picket,[21] Vilnius-Dandoy,[4] and Green-Kreuter[26] as another indicator measure to score, weight, and rank.

Regardless of the method used, the first major stage in setting community priorities is to decide upon the criteria. The framework might incl those described above or may be a composite of various approa criteria are determined, the next steps include forming a working team and/or advisory group, assembling the necessary data to conduct the prioritization process, establishing a process for stakeholder input and review, and determining a process for revisiting priorities at regular intervals. Vilnius and Dandoy recommend that a six-to-eight member group be assembled to guide the BPR process.[4] This group should include members within and outside the agency. A generic priority-setting worksheet is provided in Figure 7–2. This worksheet provides some guidance on the types of information that would typically need to be collected and summarized before a work group begins its activity.

Other Considerations and Caveats

In deciding on the use of a particular prioritization process, it important to keep several limitations in mind. No determination of public health priorities should be reduced solely to numbers; values, social justice, and the political climate all play roles. The rapid turnover in leadership within state public health agencies presents a unique challenge. The median tenure for a state public health officer is about two years,[37] which may lead to a lack of long-term focus on public health priorities. Each analytic method for prioritization has particular strengths and weaknesses. Some methods rely heavily on quantitative data, but valid and usable data can be difficult to come by, especially for smaller geographic areas such as cities or neighborhoods. It can also be difficult to identify the proper metrics for comparison of various health conditions. For example, using mortality alone would ignore the disabling burden of arthritis when it is compared to other chronic diseases. Newer measures (e.g., quality-adjusted life years) are advantageous as they are comparable across diseases and risk factors. Rankings, especially close ranks, should be assessed with caution. One useful approach is to divide a distribution of health issues into quartiles or quintiles and compare the extremes of a distribution. In addition, some key stakeholders may find that quantitative methods of prioritization fail to present a full picture, suggesting the need to use methods that combine quantitative and qualitative approaches.

INNOVATION AND CREATIVITY IN PROGRAM DEVELOPMENT

Another factor to consider in program development is innovation. Innovation has been defined as "a new method, idea, or product."[38] In most instances, there

To Use	Sample Criteria	Measure	Score	Weight[b]	Weighted Score	Priority Score
✓	(tailor to ensure criteria can be applied to all health issues being weighed)	(cite specific measure and data source if available)	(score data, assign points, or rank using identified method)	(assign value to criteria if desired)	(score multiplied by weight)	(sum of weighted scores for each criterion used)
	Prevalence					
	Mortality rate					
	Community concern					
	Lost productivity (e.g., bed-disability days)					
	Premature mortality (e.g., years of potential life lost)					
	Medical costs to treat (or community economic costs)					
	Feasibility to prevent					
	Other:					
	Other:					
	Other:					
	Other:					

FIGURE 7–2. Generic worksheet for priority setting. *Source*: Healthy People 2010 Toolkit.[7]

Note: A weight ensures that certain characteristics have a greater influence than others have in the final priority ranking. A sample formula might be: 2(Prevalence Score) + Community Concern Score + 3(Medical Cost Score) = Priority Score. In this example, the weight for prevalence is 2 and medical cost is 3. Users might enter data or assign scores (such as 1–5) for each criterion and use the formula to calculate a total score for the health event.

is a trade-off between the level to which a program is evidence-based, via the scientific literature, and the degree to which it is innovative. Consider, for example, the evidence from a review of programs that promote seat belt use to prevent motor vehicle injuries. From these, there is strong evidence that enforcement programs are effective in promoting seat belt use and hence, reducing motor vehicle injuries.[39] If you were planning to set up a program, would you follow what has already been done or try a new (and perhaps more innovative) approach? In practice, it is crucial to search for existing and new program approaches for several reasons. First, there is no guarantee that a program proven to work in one population or geographic area will yield the same results in another locality. Second, since the evidence base in many areas of public health intervention is relatively weak, a continual discovery of new and innovative approaches is crucial. And third, the development of innovative programs can be motivating for the people carrying out programs and the community members with whom they work.

Creativity in Developing Alternatives

Creativity and its role in effective decision making is not fully understood. Creativity is the process of developing original, imaginative, and innovative options.[38] To understand the role of creativity in decision making, it is helpful to know about its nature and process and the techniques for nurturing it.

Researchers have sought to understand the characteristics of creative people. There appears to be relatively little overlap between creativity and intelligence.[40] There also seems to be no difference in creativity between men and women. Several other characteristics that have been consistently associated with creativity. The typical period in the life cycle of greatest creativity appears to be between the ages of 30 and 40. It also seems that more creative people are less susceptible to social influences than those who are less creative.

The creative process has been described in four stages: preparation, incubation, insight, and verification.[41] The preparation phase is highly dependent on the education and training of the individual embarking on the creative process. Incubation usually involves a period of relaxation after a period of preparation. The human mind gathers and sorts data, and then needs time for ideas to jell. In the incubation period, it is often useful to direct energies toward some other pursuits before returning to the task at hand. In the insight phase, one gradually or rapidly, becomes aware of a new idea or approach. And finally, in the verification phase, the individual verifies the appropriateness of the idea or solution. In the business setting, this would include consumer surveys or focus groups to test the acceptance of a new product.

Within an organizational setting, a number of processes can enhance creativity in decision making. It is important to identify ways to reward creativity within an organization and to encourage the appropriate level of risk taking among employees, ensuring that individual freedom and autonomy are not unduly constrained.

Group Processes for Enhancing Creativity

In most areas of public health, important decisions are enhanced by group decision-making processes. Often in a group process, a consensus is reached on some topics. There are advantages and disadvantages to group decision-making processes (Table 7–4), but the former generally outweigh the latter.[42] Probably, the biggest advantage is that more and better information is available to inform a decision when a group is used. Additional advantages include better acceptance of the final decision, enhanced communication, and more accurate decisions. The biggest disadvantage of group decision making is that the process takes longer. However, the management literature shows that, in general, the more "person-hours" that go into a decision, the more likely it will be that the correct one emerges.[43] Other potential disadvantages include the potential for indecisiveness, compromise decisions, and domination by one individual. In addition, an outcome known as "groupthink" may result, in which the group's desire for consensus and cohesiveness overwhelms its desire to reach the best possible decision.[43, 44] One way to offset groupthink is the rotation of new members into a decision-making group.

The following sections briefly outline three popular brainstorming techniques that are useful in developing and managing an effective group process: the Delphi method, the nominal group technique, and scenario planning. Other techniques for gathering information from groups and individuals such as focus group interviews, are described in Chapter 9.

Table 7–4. Advantages and Disadvantages of Group Decision Making

Advantages	Disadvantages
More information and knowledge are available	The process takes longer and may be costlier
More alternatives are likely to be generated	Compromise decisions resulting from indecisiveness may emerge
Better acceptance of the final decision is likely, often among those who will carry out the decision	One person may dominate the group
Enhanced communication of the decision may result	"Groupthink" may occur
More accurate and creative decisions often emerge	

Source: Griffin.[42]

The Delphi Method.   The Delphi method, developed by the Rand Corporation in the 1950s, was intended as a judgment tool for prediction and forecast, involving a panel of anonymous experts to whom intensive questionnaires and feedback were given in order to obtain consensus on a particular topic.[45, 46] Although the method has been modified and used in various ways over the years, it remains a useful way to solicit and refine expert opinion. The Delphi method is most appropriate for broad, long-range issues such as strategic planning and environmental assessments. It is not feasible for routine decisions. It can be especially useful for a geographically dispersed group of experts. There are three types of Delphi: classical, policy, and decision.[47] The decision Delphi is most relevant here as it provides a forum for decisions. Panel members are not anonymous (although responses are), and the goal is a defined and supported outcome.[45, 47]

The first step in a Delphi process involves the selection of an expert panel. This panel should generally include a range of experts across the public health field, including practitioners, researchers, and funders. A panel of thirty or fewer members is often used.[48] The Delphi method may involve a series of questionnaires (by mail or e-mail) that begin more generally and, through iteration, become more specific over several weeks or months. Open-ended questions may be used in early drafts with multiple-choice responses in later versions. A flow chart for a typical Delphi process is shown in Figure 7–3.[49] Definitions of consensus within a Delphi method vary—from full consensus to majority rule—[44] and should be specified at the outset. The critical elements of a successful Delphi process include identifying an appropriate panel of experts, designing a useful set of questions, and summarizing individual input.[49]

Nominal Group Technique.   Another useful method is the nominal group technique (NGT).[50] Unlike the Delphi methods where panel members do not see each other, the NGT involves in-person interactions in the same room. However, six to ten members represent a group in name only and may not always interact as a group in a typical work setting. The NGT can be useful in generating creative and innovative alternatives and is more feasible than a Delphi Method for routine decisions. A key to a successful NGT is an experienced and competent facilitator, who assembles the group and outlines the problem to them. It is also important to outline the specific rules that the NGT will follow.[48] Often data and information, such as the prioritization data outlined in Chapter 7, will have been provided to the group in advance of the meeting. Group members are asked to write down as many alternatives as they can think of. They then take turns stating these ideas, which are recorded on a flipchart or blackboard. Discussion is limited to simple clarification. After all alternatives have been listed, each is discussed in more detail. When discussion is completed, sometimes after a series of meetings, the various alternatives are generally voted upon and rank-

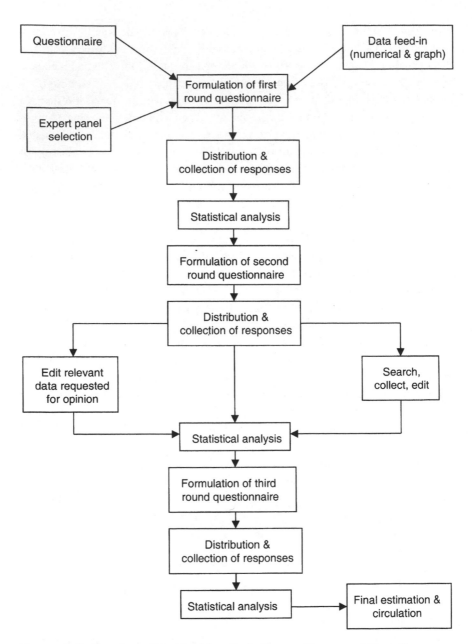

FIGURE 7–3. Flowchart of the Delphi methods (*Source*: Krueger and Casey[49]).

ordered. The primary advantage of NGT is that it can identify a large number of alternatives while minimizing the impact of group or individual opinions on the responses of individuals. The main disadvantage is that the team leader or administrator may not support the highest-ranked alternative, dampening group enthusiasm if his or her work is rejected.

Scenario Planning.   Often used in the corporate sector, scenario planning is a third useful group process for generating information for decision making. In this method, future-oriented scenarios are developed, based on how an event or system will look at some target time horizon. Scenario planning is particularly useful in an environment where there are numerous uncertainties and no clear map for the future.[51] The goal is to make decisions that are sound for all plausible futures.[52] Many characteristics and stages of scenario planning are similar to the process of environmental assessment, discussed in Chapter 4 in the context of strategic planning.

Although there are relatively few guidelines for writing scenarios, eight major stages of scenario planning have been proposed:[48]

1. Define the general area of interest or system for the scenario in operational terms
2. Establish a concrete time horizon for the scenario
3. Identify external constraints or factors that will affect the area or system of interest (e.g., social, economic, political, technological issues)
4. Describe the factors within the system that are likely to increase or decrease its chances of achieving desired goals and objectives
5. Specify the likelihood of the occurrence of facilitators to or barriers to success
6. Create one or more (often three) scenarios based on various assumptions arising in stages 3 to 5
7. Subject the scenarios to testing and review by others
8. Use the scenario for defining policy and future directions for action

Although scenarios can be very useful in planning, they can also be difficult to write. It is advisable for newcomers to scenario writing to consult someone who is experienced.

DEVELOPING AND USING ANALYTIC FRAMEWORKS

Analytic frameworks (also called logic models or causal frameworks) have benefited numerous areas of public health practice, particularly in developing and implementing clinical and community-based guidelines.[14, 53, 54] An analytic framework is a diagram that depicts the interrelationships between population characteristics, intervention components, shorter-term intervention outcomes, and longer-term public health outcomes. The major purpose of an analytic framework is to map out the linkages on which to base conclusions about intervention effectiveness.[14, 55] An underlying assumption is that various linkages represent "causal pathways," some of which are mutable and can be intervened upon. Numerous types of analytic frameworks are described in Battista and Fletcher.[56]

People designing public health interventions often have in mind an analytic framework that leads from program inputs to health outputs if the program works as intended.[57] It is important for planning and evaluation purposes that what Lipsey has termed this "small theory" of the intervention be made explicit early, often in the form of a diagram.[58] In attempting to map inputs, mediators, and outputs, it important to determine whether mediators, or constructs, lie "upstream" or "downstream" from a particular intervention.[59] As an analytic framework develops, the diagram also identifies key outcomes to be considered when formulating a data collection plan is formulated. These are then translated into public health indicators (i.e., measures of the extent to which targets in health programs are being reached[60]). Besides helping to identify key information to be collected, an analytic framework can also be viewed as a set of hypotheses about program action, including the time sequence in which program-related changes should occur; these can later guide data analysis.[57] If the program is subsequently successful in influencing outcomes at the end of this causal chain, having measures of the intermediate steps available aids interpretation by clarifying how those effects came about. Conversely, if little change in ultimate outcomes is observed, having measures of intermediate steps can help to diagnose where the causal chain was broken.[61]

Analytic frameworks can be relatively simple or complicated, with every possible relationship between risk factors, interventions, and health outcomes. A generic analytic framework is shown in Figure 7–4. A more comprehensive

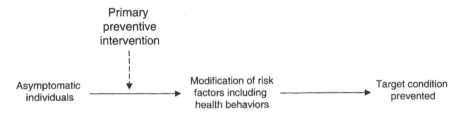

FIGURE 7–4. Generic analytic framework showing effects of primary prevention (*Source*: Battista and Fletcher[55]).

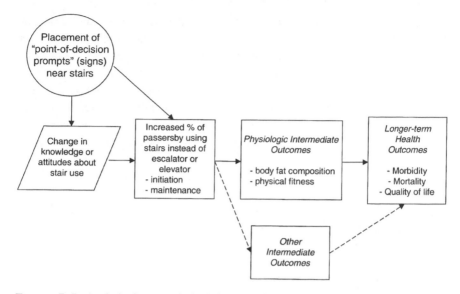

FIGURE 7–5. Analytic framework depicting the effects of point-of-decision prompts on physical activity.

approach may describe potential relationships between an intervention, intermediate outcomes, physical activity, and long-term health outcomes, as described in Figure 7–5. By developing this and related diagrams, researchers and practitioners were able to (1) indicate intervention options for changing relevant outcomes; (2) indicate categories of relevant interventions; (3) describe the outcomes that the interventions attempt to influence; and (4) indicate the types of interventions that were included in a program and those that were not.[62]

Many other examples of analytic frameworks can be found in the literature. Some of these focus on programmatic areas such as cardiovascular disease prevention,[63] drug abuse prevention,[64] and breast cancer screening.[65] Others look at mapping causal pathways in the context of program planning[23, 66] or program evaluation.[67]

Constructing Analytic Frameworks

Several approaches and sources of information are beneficial as one begins to construct an analytic framework that will map intervention options related to a particular health issue. First, a comprehensive search of the scientific literature is essential. The methods outlined in Chapter 6 form the basis for such a search. Following this search, it is likely that the practitioner will find articles that show analytic frameworks, although these are likely to vary in completeness and sophistication. Another important part in developing a framework is the identification of mutable and immutable factors along the causal pathway. A mutable factor might relate to "exposure" to a mass media campaign on a particular health issue. Conversely, an immutable factor would be a person's gender.

It is helpful to construct analytic frameworks in a professional working group. The advantages to a group process are twofold: (1) after the literature is assembled, several members of the group can independently draft initial analytic frameworks on the same topic; and (2) once initial frameworks are available, review by a small group is likely to improve the modeling. It is important to note that the construction of an analytic framework should not be viewed as a static process. As more literature and the intervention process proceeds, the framework should be modified to fit advancing knowledge of determinants. If a work group finds it too difficult to construct an analytic framework, it may indicate that the program is too complex or that its basis is not well documented.

Considering the Broad Environment

One key component in developing analytic frameworks and subsequent interventions is consideration of the "upstream" causes of poor health status. These factors are increasingly being recognized in the context of social epidemiology, that is, the socioenvironmental determinants of health, such as poverty and social isolation.[68] As shown in Table 7–5, the larger environment, including physical, social, legal, and cultural factors, needs to be fully considered as an intervention target.[69] Focus on environmental and policy factors is increasingly being recognized as an efficient and effective means for public health interventions.[69–72]

Table 7–5. Contrasting Approaches to Disease Prevention

Health Area	Individual	Environmental[a]
Smoking	Smoking cessation classes Hypnosis Nicotine patch	Cigarette taxation Clean indoor air laws Regulation of cigarette advertising
Stress	Stress reduction classes	Reduced work demands Affordable child care Crime prevention programs
Diet/weight loss	Exercise programs Cooking classes How-to-read food labels	Public transportation Affordable housing near workplace Urban public recreation areas Food security programs Food subsidy programs

Source: adapted from Yen and Syme.[69]

[a]Includes the physical, legal, social, and cultural environments.

Even though the ultimate goal is individual behavior change, environmental programs can be designed at several different levels. Social support may be built for behavior change within a worksite, and community-wide policies may be enacted to support the same health-promoting behavior. These so-called ecological interventions are discussed in more detail in Chapter 8.

SUMMARY

The public health practitioner has many tools at his or her fingertips for identifying and prioritizing program and policy options. This chapter has summarized several approaches that have proven useful for public health practitioners. As one proceeds through this process, several key points should be kept in mind:

- In public health decision making, there is seldom one "correct" answer
- Although decisions are made in the context of uncertainty and risk, classic decision theory suggests that when managers have complete information, they behave rationally
- Group decision making has advantages and disadvantages, but in most instances, the former outweighs the latter
- Priorities should not be set on quantitative factors alone
- It is often useful to apply a prioritization process on a smaller scale initially when stakes are lower
- Analytic frameworks can enhance decision making, reviews of evidence, program planning, and program evaluation

SUGGESTED READINGS AND WEBSITES

Readings

Battista RN, Fletcher SW. Making recommendations on preventive practices: methodo-
    logical issues. *American Journal of Preventive Medicine* 1988;4 Suppl:53–67.
Griffin RW. *Management.* Boston, MA: Houghton Mifflin Company, 2001.
Krueger RA, Casey MA. *Focus Groups: A Practical Guide for Applied Research.* 3rd
    ed. Thousand Oaks, CA: Sage Publications, 2000.
Vilnius D, Dandoy S. A priority rating system for public health programs. *Public Health
    Reports* 1990;105(5):463–470.

Selected Websites

Guide to Community Preventive Services <http://www.thecommunityguide.org> Under
the auspices of the U.S. Public Health Service, a Task Force on Community Preventive

Services (the Task Force) is developing a *Guide to Community Preventive Services* (the *Guide*). The *Guide* will summarize what is known about the effectiveness of population-based interventions for prevention and control.

The Centers for Disease Control and Prevention Working Group on Evaluation <http://www.cdc.gov/eval/resources.htm#journals> The Centers for Disease Control and Prevention Working Group on Evaluation has developed a comprehensive list of materials describing logic models and planning tools. The website provides various documents on line as well as links to other sites.

Healthy People 2010 Toolkit <http://www.health.gov/healthypeople/state/toolkit/> The Toolkit provides guidance, technical tools, and resources to help states, territories, and tribes develop and promote successful state-specific Healthy People 2010 plans. It can also serve as a resource for communities and other entities embarking on similar health-planning endeavors.

Models that Work Campaign <http://www.bphc.hrsa.dhhs.gov/mtw> The Models that Work Campaign identifies and promotes the replication of innovative community-based models for the delivery of primary health care to underserved and vulnerable populations. This public-private partnership, led by the Health Resources and Services Administration (HRSA), offers support to organizations and communities that are interested in increasing access to care and eliminating disparities in health status for the millions of America's neediest citizens.

Partners in Information Access for Public Health Professionals <http://www.nnlm.nlm.nih.gov/partners> A collaborative project to provide public health professionals with timely, convenient access to information resources to help them improve the health of the American public.

REFERENCES

1. Jaen CR, Stange KC, Nutting PA. The competing demands of primary care: A model for the delivery of clinical preventive services. *Journal of Family Practice* 1994;38: 166–171.
2. Stange KC, Flocke SA, Goodwin MA, Kelly RB, Zyzanski SJ. Direct observation of rates of preventive service delivery in community family practice. *Preventive Medicine* 2000;31(2 Pt 1):167–176.
3. Centers for Disease Control and Prevention. Tobacco use among middle and high school students—Florida, 1998 and 1999. *Morbidity and Mortality Weekly Report* 1999;48(12):248–253.
4. Vilnius D, Dandoy S. A priority rating system for public health programs. *Public Health Reports* 1990;105(5):463–470.
5. Green LW. Health education's contribution to public health in the twentieth century: a glimpse through health promotion's rear-view mirror. *Annual Review of Public Health* 1999;20:67–88.
6. Simon HA. *Administrative Behavior: A Study of Decision-Making Processes in Administrative Organizations*. 4th ed. New York: Free Press, 1997.
7. US Department of Health and Human Services. *Healthy People 2010 Toolkit* <www.http://www.health.gov/healthypeople/state/toolkit/>. Washington, DC: U.S. Dept. of Health and Human Services, 2001.

8. Ham C. Priority setting in health care: Learning from international experience. *Health Policy* 1997;42:49–66.

9. Eddy DM. Oregon's methods. Did cost-effectiveness analysis fail? *Journal of the American Medical Association* 1991;266(3):417–420.

10. Klevit HD, Bates AC, Castanares T, Kirk PE, Sipes-Metzler PR, Wopat R. Prioritization of health care services: a progress report by the Oregon health services commission. *Archives of Internal Medicine* 1991;151:912–916.

11. Oregon Health Services Commission. *Prioritization of Health Services. A Report to the Governor and Legislature* Portland, OR: Oregon Health Services Commission, 1995.

12. Swinburn B, Egger G, Raza F. Dissecting obesogenic environments: the development and application of a framework for identifying and prioritizing environmental interventions for obesity. *Preventive Medicine* 1999;29(6 Pt 1):563–570.

13. Canadian Task Force on the Periodic Health Examination. The periodic health examination. *Canadian Medical Association Journal* 1979;121:1193–1254.

14. Woolf SH, DiGuiseppi CG, Atkins D, Kamerow DB. Developing evidence-based clinical practice guidelines: Lessons learned by the U.S. Preventive Services Task Force. *Annual Review of Public Health* 1996;17:511–538.

15. Coffield AB, Maciosek MV, McGinnis JM, et al. Priorities among recommended clinical preventive services(1). *American Journal of Preventive Medicine* 2001;21(1): 1–9.

16. Maciosek MV, Coffield AB, McGinnis JM, et al. Methods for priority setting among clinical preventive services(1). *American Journal of Preventive Medicine* 2001;21(1): 10–19.

17. DeFriese GH, Fielding JE. Health risk appraisal in the 1990s: Opportunities, challenges, and expectations. *Annual Review of Public Health* 1990;11:401–418.

18. Yen LT, Edington DW, Witting P. Associations between health risk appraisal scores and employee medical claims costs in a manufacturing company. *American Journal of Health Promotion* 1991;6(1):46–54.

19. Patrick DL, Wickizer TM. Community and health. In: Amick BCI, Levine S, Tarlov AR, and Chapman Walsh D, eds. *Society and Health*. New York: Oxford University Press, 1995, pp. 46–92.

20. Bradford K, Simoes E. *A Model for Prioritization of Public Health Programs* Jefferson City, MO: Missouri Department of Health, January 16, 2000.

21. Hanlon J, Pickett G. *Public Health Administration and Practice*. Santa Clara, CA: Times Mirror/Mosby College Publishing, 1982.

22. Meltzer M, Teutsch SM. Setting priorities for health needs and managing resources. In: Stroup DF, Teutsch SM, eds. *Statistics in Public Health. Quantitative Approaches to Public Health Problems*. New York: Oxford University Press, 1998, pp. 123–149.

23. Simons-Morton BG, Greene WH, Gottlieb NH. *Introduction to Health Education and Health Promotion*. 2nd ed. Prospect Heights, IL: Waveland Press, 1995.

24. Zaza S, Lawrence RS, Mahan CS, et al. Scope and organization of the Guide to Community Preventive Services. *American Journal of Preventive Medicine* 2000; 18(1S):27–34.

25. Hahn RA, Teutsch SM, Rothenberg RB, Marks JS. Excess deaths from nine chronic diseases in the United States, 1986. *Journal of the American Medical Association* 1990;264(20):2654–2659.

26. Green LW, Kreuter MW. Commentary on the emerging Guide to Community Pre-

ventive Services from a health promotion perspective. *American Journal of Preventive Medicine* 2000;18(1S):7–9.

27. Missouri Department of Health. *The Missouri Foundation for Health. Report to the Board* Jefferson City, MO: Missouri Department of Health, July 2001.

28. Wolf AM, Colditz GA. Current estimates of the economic cost of obesity in the United States. *Obesity Research* 1998;6(2):97–106.

29. Basu S, Landis JR. Model-based estimation of population attributable risk under cross-sectional sampling. *American Journal of Epidemiology* 1995;142(12):1338–1343.

30. Bruzzi P, Green SB, Byar DP, Brinton LA, Schairer C. Estimating the population attributable risk for multiple risk factors using case-control data. *American Journal of Epidemiology* 1985;122(5):904–914.

31. Brownson RC, Remington PL, Davis JR, eds. *Chronic Disease Epidemiology and Control* 2nd ed. Washington, DC: American Public Health Association, 1998.

32. Powell KE, Blair SN. The public health burdens of sedentary living habits: theoretical but realistic estimates. *Medicine and Science in Sports and Exercise* 1994;26(7):851–856.

33. Shinton R. Lifelong exposures and the potential for stroke prevention: the contribution of cigarette smoking, exercise, and body fat. *Journal of Epidemiology and Community Health* 1997;51(2):138–143.

34. Carvette ME, Hayes EB, Schwartz RH, Bogdan GF, Bartlett NW, Graham LB. Chronic disease mortality in Maine: Assessing the targets for prevention. *Journal of Public Health Management and Practice* 1996;2(3):25–31.

35. Iademarco MF, Biek RW, Fields L, Brownson RC. Assessing excess deaths in St. Louis, Missouri: 1980 to 1994. *Journal of Public Health Management Practice* 1999;5(6):41–54.

36. Hoffarth S, Brownson RC, Gibson BB, Sharp DJ, Schramm W, Kivlaham C. Preventable mortality in Missouri: Excess deaths from nine chronic diseases, 1979–1991. *Missouri Medicine* 1993;90(6):279–282.

37. Gilbert B, Moos MK, Miller CA. State level decision-making for public health: The status of boards of health. *Journal of Public Health Policy* 1982♂rch:51–61.

38. Jewell EJ, Abate F, eds. *The New Oxford American Dictionary*. New York: Oxford University Press, 2001.

39. Centers for Disease Control and Prevention. Motor-vehicle occupant injury: Strategies for increasing use of child safety seats, increasing use of safety belts, and reducing alcohol-impaired driving. A report of the Task Force on Community Preventive Services. *Morbidity and Mortality Weekly Report* 2001;50(RR-7):1–16.

40. Anastasi A, Schaefer CE. Note on the concepts of creativity and intelligence. *Journal of Creative Behavior* 1971;5(2):113–116.

41. Busse TV, Mansfield RS. Theories of the creative process: a review and a perspective. *Journal of Creative Behavior* 1980;4(2):91–103.

42. Griffin RW. *Management*. Boston, MA: Houghton Mifflin Company, 2001.

43. Von Bergen CW, Kirk R. Groupthink. When too many heads spoil the decision. *Management Review* 1978;67(3):44–49.

44. Janis IL. *Groupthink*. Boston: Houghton Mifflin, 1982.

45. Crisp J, Pelletier D, Duffield C, Adams A, Nagy S. The Delphi Method? *Nursing Research* 1997;46(2):116–118.

46. Dalkey N, Helmer O. An experimental application of the Delphi method to the use of experts. *Management Science* 1963;9:458–467.
47. Rauch W. The decision Delphi. *Technological Forecasting and Social Change* 1979; 15:159–169.
48. Witkin BR, Altschuld JW. *Conducting and Planning Needs Assessments. A Practical Guide*. Thousand Oaks, CA: Sage Publications, 1995.
49. Krueger RA, Casey MA. *Focus Groups: A Practical Guide for Applied Research*. 3rd ed. Thousand Oaks, CA: Sage Publications, 2000.
50. Delbecq AL, Van de Ven AH. *Group Techniques for Program Planning*. Glenview, IL: Scott, Foresman, 1975.
51. Ginter PM, Swayne LM, Duncan WJ. *Strategic Management of Health Care Organizations*. 4th ed. Malden, MA: Blackwell Publishers Inc., 2002.
52. Schwartz P. *The Art of the Long View. Paths to Strategic Insight for Yourself and Your Company*. New York: Currency Doubleday, 1991.
53. Pappaioanou M, Evans C. Developing a guide to community preventive services: A U.S. Public Health Service initiative. *Journal of Public Health Management and Practice* 1998;4:48–54.
54. US Preventive Services Task Force. *Guide to Clinical Preventive Services*. 2nd ed. Baltimore: Williams & Wilkins, 1996.
55. Woolf SH. An organized analytic framework for practice guideline development: Using the analytic logic as a guide for reviewing evidence, developing recommendations, and explaining the rationale. In: McCormick KA and Moore SR, eds. *Methodology Perpectives*. Rockville, MD: Agency for Health Care Policy Research, 1994, pp. 105–113.
56. Battista RN, Fletcher SW. Making recommendations on preventive practices: Methodological issues. *American Journal of Preventive Medicine* 1988;4 Suppl:53–67.
57. Koepsell TD. Epidemiologic issues in the design of community intervention trials. In: Brownson RC and Pettiti DB, eds. *Applied Epidemiology: Theory to Practice*. New York: Oxford University Press, 1998, pp. 177–211.
58. Lipsey MW. Theory as Method: Small Theories of Treatment. In: Sechrest L, Perrin E, and Bunker J, eds. *Research Methodology: Strengthening Causal Interpretations of Nonexperimental Data*. Vol DHHS Pub. No. (PHS) 90–3454. Washington, DC: Government Printing Office, 1990.
59. MacKinnon DP, Dwyer JH. Estimating mediated effects in prevention studies. *Evaluation Research* 1993;12:144–158.
60. World Health Organization. *Health program evaluation. Guiding principles for its application in the managerial process for national development Health for All* Series, No.6. Geneva, Switzerland: World Health Organization; 1981.
61. Koepsell TD, Wagner EH, Cheadle AC, et al. Selected methodological issues in evaluating community-based health promotion and disease prevention programs. *Annual Review of Public Health* 1992;13:31–57.
62. Briss PA, Zaza S, Pappaioanou M, et al. Developing an evidence-based Guide to Community Preventive Services—methods. The Task Force on Community Preventive Services. *American Journal of Preventive Medicine* 2000;18(1 Suppl):35–43.
63. Goodman RM, Wheeler FC, Lee PR. Evaluation of the Heart to Heart Project: Lessons from a community-based chronic disease prevention project. *American Journal of Health Promotion* 1995;9:443–455.
64. Pentz MA, Dwyer JH, MacKinnon DP, et al. A multicommunity trial for primary

prevention of adolescent drug abuse. Effects on drug use prevalence. *Journal of the American Medical Association* 1989;261:3259–3266.

65. Worden JK, Mickey RM, Flynn BS, et al. Development of a community breast screening promotion program using baseline data. *Preventive Medicine* 1994;23:267–275.

66. Green LW, Kreuter MW. *Health Promotion Planning: An Educational and Ecological Approach* 3rd ed. Mountain View, CA: Mayfield, 1999.

67. Centers for Disease Control and Prevention. Framework for program evaluation in public health. *Morbidity and Mortality Weekly Report* 1999;48(RR-11):1–40.

68. Berkman LF, Kawachi I. A historical framework for social epidemiology. In: Berkman LF and Kawachi I, eds. *Social Epidemiology*. New York: Oxford University Press; 2000:3–12.

69. Yen IH, Syme SL. The social environment and health: A discussion of the epidemiologic literature. *Annual Review of Public Health* 1999;20:287–308.

70. Brownson RC, Newschaffer CJ, Ali-Abarghoui F. Policy research for disease prevention: Challenges and practical recommendations. *American Journal of Public Health* 1997;87(5):735–739.

71. McKinlay JB. The promotion of health through planned sociopolitical change: Challenges for research and policy. *Social Science and Medicine* 1993;36(2):109–117.

72. Schmid TL, Pratt M, Howze E. Policy as intervention: environmental and policy approaches to the prevention of cardiovascular disease. *American Journal of Public Health* 1995;85(9):1207–1211.

8

Developing an Action Plan and Implementing Interventions

> Even if you're on the right track, you'll get run over if you just sit there.
>
> —Will Rogers

Once a particular program or policy has been identified, sound planning techniques can ensure that the program is implemented effectively. It can be argued that planning is the most fundamental and most important administrative function.[1] In the context of community change, sound action planning is one of the key factors predicting success.[2] The focus of this chapter is on *action planning*, i.e., planning for a defined program or policy with specific, time-dependent outcomes, as compared with ongoing planning that is a regular function within an organization.

Effective action plans have several key characteristics.[1,3] First, they have clear aims and objectives. Second, the roles and responsibilities of important stakeholders are clarified and respected. Third, there are clear mechanisms for accountability. Fourth, the plans are comprehensive in that they utilize multiple intervention tactics (communication, behavioral, policy, regulatory, environmental). Such comprehensiveness includes a listing of all possible action steps and changes. This is an area where a sound analytic framework (see Chapter 7) can be especially useful in describing potential interventions and their effects. The plan must also have mechanisms for evaluation. Finally, an action plan needs to be current and based on the latest scientific evidence.

To cover some essential issues for successful action planning, this chapter is organized in five main sections, designed to highlight ecological frameworks, give examples of behavioral science models that can increase the likelihood of carrying out effective interventions, review key principles of planning, outline steps in action planning, and describe important aspects of coalition-based interventions.

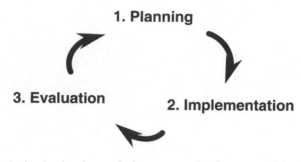

FIGURE 8–1. A simple planning cycle for program development and implementation.

BACKGROUND

Solid action planning takes into account essentially all of the issues and approaches covered elsewhere in this book. For example, let's assume we are broadly concerned with the public health needs of a community. Early in the process, we have examined epidemiologic data and conducted prioritization to establish the basis for selecting which health issues to address. Systematic reviews of the literature and cost-effectiveness studies would have assisted us in determining possible intervention approaches and in "selling" a program to policy makers. Through our needs and resource assessment (or "diagnosis") we have engaged multiple stakeholders and community members in the process.[4, 5] And we have used a wide range of local data sets to guide our decision-making process. All of these earlier steps need to be kept in mind in the process of designing and implementing program strategies. In addition, program monitoring and evaluation (see Chapter 9) are essential in determining the impact(s) of a program or policy.

In simple terms, program or policy development consists of planning, implementation, and evaluation (Figure 8–1). The earlier chapters in this book described the tools, strategies, and steps needed to determine which issue(s) should be addressed via a public health intervention. In this chapter, our attention turns to the matter of implementation: "What specific actions can we take that are most likely to yield the change in health and/or health behaviors we seek?"

ECOLOGICAL FRAMEWORKS

Ecological frameworks have been applied across a variety of settings and public health issues. An ecological framework is a useful way to organize objectives and intervention approaches (Table 8–1). In general, the use of ecological models has outpaced evaluation studies in the attempt to document the effectiveness of

Table 8–1. Summary of Objectives and Intervention Approaches across Levels of an Ecological Framework

	Individual	Interpersonal	Organizational	Community	Health Policy
Objectives address:	Knowledge	Programs	Programs	Programs	Ordinances
	Attitudes	Practices	Practices	Practices	Regulations
	Behavior	Social support	Policies	Policies	Laws
		Social networks	Built environment	Built environment	Policies
Approaches:	Information	Develop new social ties	Organizational change	Social change	Political action
	Education	Lay health advisors	Networking	Media advocacy	Lobbying
	Training	Peer support groups	Organizational development	Coalition building	Media advocacy
	Counseling		Environmental changes	Community development	Policy advocacy
				Environmental changes	Coalition building

Source: adapted from Simons-Morton et al.[31]

these frameworks and the mechanisms by which changes in health behaviors occur.[6, 7] As shown in Box 8–1, an ecological framework can be modified and adapted for complex issues such as HIV prevention.[8] A study of forty-four health promotion programs in Canada found that most programs (68%) were limited to one intervention setting, such as an organization, and only two of forty-four programs occurred in four settings.[9] We believe that a developing literature shows that action planning will be improved if it is based on an ecological framework.

Ecological frameworks suggest that it is important to address individual, interpersonal, organizational, community (social and economic), and health policy factors because of the effect these factors have on individual behavior change and because of their direct effect on health.[10] At the extremes, an ecological framework has two main options: changing people or changing the environment.[6] In fact, the most effective interventions probably act at multiple levels since communities are made up of individuals who interact in a variety of social networks and within a particular context. The literature review, assessment of needs and resources, and evaluation of available data sets can help to guide which level (or levels) of the ecological framework is the appropriate level for intervention.

Several variations of an ecological framework have been proposed.[11–14] Adapted from McLeroy and colleagues,[11] five levels of intervention are possible:

1. Individual factors—characteristics of the individual such as knowledge, attitudes, skills, and a person's developmental history
2. Interpersonal factors—formal and informal social networks and social support systems, including family and friends
3. Organizational factors—social institutions, organizational characteristics, and rules or regulations for operation
4. Community factors—relationships between organizations, economic forces, the physical environment, and cultural variables that shape behavior
5. Health policy factors—local, state, and national laws, rules, and regulations

Programs focused on changing *individual* behavior may provide information and teach skills to enable individuals to change their behaviors. These programs may focus on changing knowledge, attitudes, beliefs, and behaviors. Various theories can be useful in directing practitioners to specific strategies that are appropriate to use in changing individual behavior (as described later in this chapter.) Some theories, such as the stages-of-change theory, suggest that different approaches are likely to be more or less useful, depending on the individual's readiness for change.[15–17]

To address *interpersonal* factors, many programs include strategies to

Box 8–1. An Ecological Approach to HIV Prevention among Asian and Pacific Islander American Men

In the United States, the incidence of AIDS is increasing at a higher rate among Asian and Pacific Islander men who have sex with men (MSM) than among Caucasian MSM. To work out an approach that would be more effective in preventing HIV among Asian and Pacific Islander American men, Choi and colleagues[8] reviewed five major models of health behavior change: the health belief model, the theory of reasoned action, social learning theory, diffusion theory, and the AIDS risk reduction model. The authors concluded that these five models did not adequately address environmental influences on HIV transmission. Recent empirical evidence suggests that interventions need to target both individuals and environmental determinants of HIV transmission. To reach multiple levels of HIV prevention, Choi et al. proposed an ecological framework of three levels as a potentially useful method of organizing interventions:

- Individual: programs to enhance the ability to accept his ethnic or sexual identity
- Interpersonal: interventions to target families, enhancing communication about sex in families with gay children
- Community: mass media campaigns to educate the community about sexual diversity and to promote positive images of ethnically diverse men in the gay community

Clear evaluation strategies must be used to examine the effects of HIV prevention programs that target multiple levels of an ecological framework.

strengthen social support. As described by Israel,[18] these programs may act in various ways. For example, programs may attempt to strengthen existing networks by working with families and friends. Alternatively, programs may develop new network ties through social support groups or may enhance the capacity of natural helpers, such as people in positions of respect in a community, to provide health-related information and assistance. A program aimed at strengthening existing social networks to enhance individual behavior change might invite family members to join exercise facilities or take cooking classes together. Programs may also seek to enhance the total network through lay health advisors.[18] According to Israel, lay health advisors are "lay people to whom others normally turn to for advice, emotional support and tangible aid."[19] Lay health advisors may provide information on specific health risks or behaviors or on services available to address various health needs. They may also assist clients in improving their communication skills, or establish linkages with health and human service agencies for efficient and appropriate referral.[20] In some instances, building social ties may be a secondary aim of programs that primarily focus on other types of community-based activities.

At the *organizational* level, characteristics of an organization can be used to support positive behavior change. One may attempt to change the organization itself, and organizations may be an ideal setting for "diffusion" of interventions that have proven useful in other settings.[11] Organizations such as day care facilities, schools, and worksites are particularly important for enhancing public health because people spend one-third to one-half of their lives in such settings.[11]

Public health programs may also attempt to create changes in *community* and *health policy* factors. These efforts often focus on creating changes in community structures, processes, and policies. Changes in community structures or processes could include development of community parks, libraries, or educational facilities and may also involve changes in decision-making structures to incorporate points of view that were previously unheard. In terms of policy changes, these programs may, for example, focus on creating smoke-free public places to support changes in individual smoking behavior and attempt to alter community norms around smoking.[21] Alternately, efforts may be focused on creating policy changes in other social, community, or economic factors such as housing, jobs, education, and the environment.[22] Existing channels in a community may be useful for intervention delivery. Churches, for example, have been shown to be useful for community health programs.[23] They provide easy access for community needs assessments. Second, the church community is defined by its religious belief system, including beliefs and attitudes about health behaviors. And third, churches are frequently the community's center. Since they may already identify at-risk members of the congregation, provide referrals to services, and provide some health services themselves, they are well placed to serve as a headquarters for health programming.

Ecological frameworks suggest that individual, interpersonal, organizational, community, and health policy factors are interrelated, and programs that address one level are likely to enhance outcomes at the other levels.[7] Levels of the ecological framework are overlapping. A new health policy might be implemented in a worksite that employs a significant proportion of a town's population, and this might result in a change in social norms throughout a community. It is also important to note that ecological frameworks are useful whether the program is categorical (focused on a particular disease process) or a broadly defined community program like community development. Programs that focus on a disease category such as breast cancer and receive categorical funding to change individual behavior (e.g., getting mammograms) will enhance their ability to influence this behavior if they consider the impact of interpersonal and organizational factors and intervene accordingly. This may entail providing low or no cost mammograms, changing the policy in the state so that more women are eligible for low- or no-cost mammograms, developing a lay health advisor approach to enhance breast cancer screening, or changing transportation systems to give women better access to screening and treatment services. These programmatic activities may occur simultaneously or sequentially.

THE ROLE OF THEORY IN CREATING PROGRAMS AND POLICIES

The effectiveness of public health interventions can be enhanced by the use of systematic planning frameworks (e.g., logic models) and theory (e.g., the "transtheoretical model," social learning theory, policy development theories).[24, 25]

Logic models, or analytic frameworks, were described in Chapter 7. When used in program planning, a logic model outlines specific activities and explains how they will lead to the accomplishment of objectives and how these objectives will enhance the likelihood of accomplishing program goals.[26, 27] For example, a logic model lays out what the program participants will do (attend an educational session on breast cancer screening at their church), what it will lead to (increased knowledge regarding risk factors for breast cancer and specific methods of breast cancer screening), which will in turn will have an impact (increase breast cancer screening rates), with the intention that this will therefore produce a long-term outcome (decreased morbidity due to breast cancer). Several authors have conceptualized this process somewhat differently, yet the overall intent is that the program or policy be laid out with specific objectives and activities that are expected to have an impact on clearly delineated outcomes, both near- and long-term.

The specific program or policy activities to be developed should be determined by their ability to meet the objectives outlined in the logic model and should be based on sound theories or models of behavior and community change. Theory helps practitioners ask the right questions, and effective action planning assists them in zeroing in on elements that relate to a specific problem.[6] Planning frameworks and theories help us understand why people are not living more health-promoting lifestyles or following medical advice, what needs to be done before developing and organizing a program or policy, and what should be monitored or measured during evaluation.[28]

A theory is a set of interrelated concepts, definitions, and propositions that presents a systematic view of events or situations by specifying relations among variables in order to explain and predict events or situations.[28] Theories and models explain behavior and suggest ways to achieve behavior change.[28] As noted by Bandura, in advanced disciplines like mathematics, theories integrate laws; whereas, in newer fields such as public health or behavioral science, theories describe or specify the determinants governing the phenomena of interest.[29] Moreover, in terms of action planning, theory can point to important intervention strategies. For example, if perceptions are considered important in maintaining behavior, then it will be crucial to include some strategies to alter perceptions; whereas, if skills are considered important to change behavior, then some strategy to alter skills must be included in the intervention. While it is not possible to provide a summary of all of the theories that might be used in developing programmatic and policy strategies, some discussion of how theory can be translated to practice is important. Therefore, a brief overview of two individual-level theories is presented below with a focus on how the constructs in the theories guide specific action strategies.

Individual-Level Theories

Based on a review conducted by Glanz and colleagues of twenty-four journals in health education, medicine, and behavioral sciences, from 1992 to 1994, the most commonly used theories of how to change individual behavior are: the Health Belief Model, the Social Cognitive Theory/Social Learning Theory, self-efficacy, the Theory of Reasoned Action/Theory of Planned Behavior, and the Stages-of-Change/Transtheoretical Model.[28] It is important to note that many of the constructs of the various theories overlap, sometimes with slightly differing terminology.[30] For example, outcome expectations within the Social Learning Theory relate to an individual's belief about the likelihood that a specific behavior will lead to a particular outcome.[29] This relates closely to behavioral beliefs within the Theory of Reasoned Action/Theory of Planned Behavior. The following sections briefly describe two common behavior-change theories: the Health Belief Model and the Transtheoretical Model. Readers are referred elsewhere[25, 29] for more detailed descriptions of various theories.

The Health Belief Model. The Health Belief Model (HBM) may be the most widely used and best known of theoretical frameworks in health behavior change.[31, 32] This model was developed in the 1950s, based on experience in a screening program for tuberculosis. The HBM is a "value expectancy theory," i.e., in the context of health-related behavior, individuals hold both the desire to avoid illness or to get well (a value) and the belief that a specific health action will prevent illness (expectancy). The expectancy can be further defined in terms of an individual's estimate of personal susceptibility to and severity of an illness and perceived benefits and barriers to action. The HBM also emphasized the role of perception in behavior change.[31] According to the HBM, an individual's cognitions or perceptions determine behavior.

The HBM recognizes four important categories of beliefs that are important in health behavior change:

1. Perceived susceptibility—an individual's opinion of the likelihood of getting a certain health condition
2. Perceived severity—an individual's opinion of how serious a condition and its sequelae are

3. Perceived benefits—an individual's opinion of the advantages of the advised action to reduce risk
4. Perceived barriers—an individual's opinion of the tangible and psychological costs of the advised action

Two more recently described constructs include cues to action (strategies to activate one's readiness) and self-efficacy (one's confidence in one's ability to take action).[32] The HBM can be useful in action planning,[33] since it provides an outline of some essential factors involved in individual behavior change and suggests that cognitions and perceptions are important in helping individuals to change their behavior.

The Transtheoretical Model (Stages of Change).   The Transtheoretical Model was developed to integrate principles across major theories of health behavior change, hence the name *trans*theoretical.[15, 17] It suggests that people move through one of five "stages" and that health behavior change is an evolving process that can be more effectively achieved if the intervention of choice matches the stage of readiness to change behavior. In the following descriptions, the time frame has been defined for some behaviors such as smoking cessation but is less established for others such as beginning a physical activity program. The five stages are as follows:

1. Precontemplation—No intention to change behavior in the foreseeable future (usually measured as the next six months); unaware of the risk; deny the consequences of risk behavior.
2. Contemplation—Aware that a problem exists; Seriously thinking about overcoming it, but have not yet made a commitment to take action; Anticipated that he/she will take action in the next six months.
3. Preparation—Intend to take action in the near future and may have taken some inconsistent action in the past. Time frame for taking action usually measured as within the next month.
4. Action—Modify behavior, experiences, or environment to overcome problems; behavior change is relatively recent (generally, within the past six months).
5. Maintenance—Work to prevent relapse and maintain the behavior over a long period of time (usually from six months to five years).
   [In addition, a sixth stage (Termination) applies to some addictive behaviors. In Termination, the individual is certain that he/she will not return to the unhealthy behavior, even in times of stress as a way of coping.[17]]

Numerous studies have examined the effectiveness of staged materials in health education interventions. In general, studies find that stage-tailored mate-

Box 8–2. Stages of Change Intervention for Promoting Fruit and Vegetable Consumption in Worksites

The *5-a-Day for Better Health* program originally developed by the California Department of Health Services, was designed to increase fruit and vegetable consumption in line with year 2000 and 2010 health objectives. A related project, *Seattle 5-a-Day*, was carried out at a total of twenty-eight worksites that were randomized to either intervention or control.[34] The intervention occurred at the individual and organizational levels and was developed around the stages-of-change behavioral model. The project emphasized employee involvement in order to build ownership for the project. To move participants from precontemplation to contemplation, early phase activities focused on raising general awareness and motivating thinking about change. A "teaser" campaign was used to alert employees that something new was coming soon to the worksite. In the second phase, events were held to move participants from contemplation to preparation. In the final phase, the goal was movement from preparation to action via skill building and worksite changes in the cafeteria, such as point-of-purchase displays. Based on data collected via a food frequency questionnaire at baseline and a two-year follow-up, a net intervention effect of 0.3 daily servings of fruits and vegetables was shown. It appears that the stages-of-change model formed a useful framework for this intervention. This relatively simple intervention approach could be applied in worksites with cafeterias.

rials are more effective than generic materials in moving individuals through the various stages. In other words, at the early stages, cognitive change strategies are more likely to be helpful in moving individuals to the next stage, while in later stages, skill building may be useful. An example of a stage-based intervention for dietary change is shown in Box 8–2.[34] Researchers are also studying the utility of the Transtheoretical Model beyond the individual level. Their research is focusing on such issues as the potential interactions between social support and stages of change, the staging of organizations in the change process, and attempts to match health policy initiatives with the readiness to change in a community.[17]

COMMON PRINCIPLES ACROSS PLANNING FRAMEWORKS

Numerous frameworks for planning have been proposed over the past few decades. Among the earliest approaches was a simple program evaluation and review technique (PERT) chart. As described by Breckon and colleagues,[35] this was a graphically displayed time line for the tasks necessary in the development and implementation of a public health program. Subsequent approaches have divided program development into various phases, including needs assessment, goal setting, problem definition, plan design, implementation, and evaluation.[31] There are numerous other planning frameworks that have proven useful for various intervention settings and approaches. Among them are

- The Planned Approach to Community Health (PATCH)[24]
- Predisposing, Reinforcing and Enabling Constructs in Educational/environmental Diagnosis and Evaluation, with its implementation phase: Policy, Regulatory and Organizational Constructs in Educational and Environmental Development (PRECEDE-PROCEED)[36]
- Multilevel Approach to Community Health (MATCH)[31]

Each of these frameworks has been used to plan and implement successful programs. The PRECEDE-PROCEED model alone has generated in excess of 1,500 documented health promotion applications in a variety of settings and across multiple health problems. Rather than providing a review of each of these planning frameworks, we have extracted those planning principles that appear to be crucial to the success of interventions in community settings and are common to each framework. Those principles include the following:[37]

1. Data should guide the development of programs. Elsewhere in this book, we describe many types and sources of data that are useful in summarizing a community's health status, needs, and assets in the community to make changes.
2. Community members should participate in the process. As discussed in Chapter 4, active participation by a range of community members in setting priorities, planning interventions, and making decisions enhances the viability and staying power of many public health programs.
3. Participants should develop a comprehensive intervention strategy. Based on a participatory process, community members are encouraged to develop comprehensive intervention strategies across multiple sectors, including mass media, schools, and health care facilities. This relates closely to a socioecological approach, described above.
4. The community capacity for health promotion should be increased. A systematic planning process can be repeated to address various health priorities. Such an approach aims to increase capacity to improve public health by enhancing the community's skills in health planning and health promotion.
5. Evaluation should emphasize feedback and program improvement. Sound evaluation improves program delivery and for such, timely feedback to the community is essential.

Table 8–2. Steps in Designing a Successful Public Health Intervention

1. Review health data; determine contributing factors
2. Identify existing programs and policies
3. Obtain support in the setting for intervention (e.g., community, health care, schools)
4. Involve the target group
5. Determine potential barriers and solutions
6. Use evidence to select effective intervention strategies
7. Set specific objectives
8. Develop the evaluation plan
9. Develop work plan and timetables
10. Assess resource needs
11. Identify and train workers
12. Pilot test intervention and evaluation
13. Monitor and evaluate program or policy
14. Use evaluation results

Source: adapted from *The Planned Approach to Community Health* (PATCH)[37] and Davis et al.[38]

A STEPWISE APPROACH TO SUCCESSFUL ACTION PLANNING

The preceding frameworks and keys to intervention success help to form a stepwise framework for successful action planning (Table 8–2).[37, 38] Within this fourteen-step approach, previous chapters have primarily dealt with the first six issues; this section will highlight steps seven through eleven; Chapter 9 addresses evaluation issues in detail. As noted earlier, effective implementation requires sound management skills, ranging from strategic planning and effective fiscal oversight to human resources management. While it is beyond the scope of this chapter or book to review each management or implementation issue in detail, we will briefly cover several key issues that are essential for any successful program.

Making the Correct Managerial Decisions

Developing and implementing effective programs and policies requires sound management skills. Public health management is the process of constructing, implementing, and evaluating organized responses to a health problem or a series of interrelated health problems.[39] One of the goals of an evidence-based process is to make rational and well-grounded decisions—a management function. Important decisions always carry some element of risk. Sound management and planning is iterative, generally does not lead to a single option, and does not eliminate the risk of making poor judgments.[39] In addition, complex public health problems are rarely resolved by implementing a single program or policy.

Rather, change often requires a set of actions. The goal of action planning is, therefore, to maximize the chances of efficient use of resources and effective delivery of programs and policies. Previous chapters provide data to help guide the managerial decisions regarding *which* program or policy to implement. This chapter deals with implementation—the process of putting a program or policy into effect. In implementation, one seeks to accomplish the setting up, management, and execution of the program.[1]

Setting Objectives

It is essential to understand the components of sound program objectives.[1, 31, 39] This is of paramount importance because sound planning and evaluation are based on a series of objectives. A rigorous commitment to setting and monitoring objectives builds quality control into a program or policy and allows for mid-course corrections via process evaluation (see Chapter 9). An intervention objective should include a clear identification of the health issue or risk factor being addressed, the at-risk population being addressed, the current status of the health issue or risk factor in the at-risk population, and the desired outcome of the intervention. A clearly defined objective can guide both the development of intervention content and the selection of appropriate communication channels. It also facilitates the development of quantitative evaluation measures that can be used to monitor the success of the intervention and to identify opportunities for improvement. Importantly, a clearly defined objective will improve the coordination of activities among the various partners participating in the intervention.

Several aspects of sound objective-setting have been described:[1, 40]

- There must be sound scientific evidence to support the objectives.
- The result to be achieved should be important and understandable to a broad audience.
- Objectives should be prevention-oriented and should address health improvements that can be achieved through population-based and/or health-service interventions.
- Objectives should drive action and suggest a set of interim steps (intermediate indicators) that will achieve the proposed targets within the specified time frame.
- The language of objectives should be precise, avoiding use of general or vague verbs.
- Objectives should be measurable and may include a range of measures—health outcomes, behavioral risk factors, health service indicators, or assessments

Table 8–3. Examples of Objectives and Their Linkages to Action Strategies

Level/Organization	Objective	Action Strategies
National/ U.S. Department of Health and Human Services	Increase the proportion of persons aged 2 years and older who consume at least two daily servings of fruit. Increase the proportion of persons aged 2 years and older who consume at least three daily servings of vegetables, with at least one-third being dark green or orange vegetables.	Convene a national steering committee that develops and implements a multipronged National Strategic Plan that uses social marketing tools, is integrated across state, regional and local levels, and employs a public/private partnership approach at all levels.
State/Minnesota Department of Health	By the year 2004, increase by 10% the number of children, adolescents and adults who consume five or more servings of fruits and vegetables daily, six or more servings of beans and grains daily, and adequate intakes of calcium.	Conduct public information campaigns and events to promote healthy, low-fat eating, including promoting the daily consumption of five or more servings of fruits and vegetables, adequate calcium intake, and healthy weight management.

of community capacity. They should count assets and achievements and look to the positive.

• Specific timetables for completion of objectives should be described.

Table 8–3 presents examples of sound objectives from national and state governmental sectors. These are drawn from the strategic plans and other planning materials of the programs noted.

Developing the Workplan and Timetables

A detailed implementation plan will enhance the chances of a successful program. Defining lines of authority and communication is crucial for a community-based program in which numerous activities may occur simultaneously. In conjunction, the time frame for the program or policy should be carefully mapped in the form of a time line. For externally funded projects like grants and contracts, this time line corresponds to the funding period. A time line is a graphic presentation of information, including a list of all activities (or milestones) and designating when they are to be accomplished. Basic time line construction includes the following:[1]

1. A complete listing of activities, grouped by major categories
2. Ascertaining which activities need to be done first

Activity	Month												
	1	2	3	4	5	6	7	8	9	10	11	12
Administration												
• Hire and train staff	x	x										
• Assemble research team	x	x										
• Conduct staff meetings	x	x	x	x	x	x	x	x	x	x	x	x
• Oversee and manage budget	x	x	x	x	x	x	x	x	x	x	x	x
Intervention Development & Implementation												
• Conduct focus groups to refine interventions			x	x								
• Pilot test interventions					x	x						
• Finalize interventions and begin delivery							x	x	x			
Data Collection & Evaluation												
• Test and finalize questionnaires					x	x						
• Review pilot data and refine data collection approaches						x	x					
• Conduct process evaluation									x	x	x	x
• Conduct impact evaluation									x	x	x	x
Analysis and Dissemination (all year two or year three activities)												
• Edit data and conduct data entry												
• Refine and conduct analyzes												
• Write rough draft and final project report												
• Present findings at regional and national meetings												

*Only year one is displayed as an example.

FIGURE 8–2. Example time line for implementation of a public health intervention. (Only one year is displayed as an example.)

3. Determining how long each activity will take
4. Determining when each and every activity is to begin and finish
5. Establishing the time units that are most appropriate (weeks, months, years)

An sample time line is shown in Figure 8–2. Although there are many ways to organize a time line, this example groups activities into four main categories: (1) administration; (2) intervention development and implementation; (3) data collection and evaluation; and (4) analysis and dissemination. For internal purposes it is useful to add another component to this time line—that of the personnel intended to carry out each task. Doing this in conjunction with the time line will allow for assessment of work load and personnel needs at various times throughout the proposed project. Another important component of program delivery is the assessment of program implementation: How well was the program delivered?[41] These issues are covered in more detail in chapter 9 within the context of process evaluation.

Assessing Resource Needs

A manager needs to determine the resources required to implement a particular program or policy. Resources can be grouped into five general areas:

1. Available funds: How many direct funds are available? What are the sources? Are there limitations on how and when funds can be spent? Are funds internal or external to your program or agency? Are there "in kind" funds?

2. Personnel: How many and what types of personnel are needed? What type of training will be needed for program staff? What personnel do collaborating organizations bring to the project?
3. Equipment and Materials: What types of equipment and supplies are needed for the program? Are there certain pieces of equipment that can be obtained "in-kind" from participating partners?
4. Facilities: For some types of interventions, is significant infrastructure needed (such as clinics, hospitals, or mobile vans)?

Line Item	Internal Resources (new budget allocation)	Internal In-Kind (reallocation of existing resources)	External Resources (grants, contracts, other public or private sources)	External In-Kind (donated services or non-financial resources)
Personnel (staff or contractors) *Examples*: Coordinator Data manager Health educator Evaluator Administrative support staff Technical support/consultants Subject matter experts Meeting facilitators Graphic designer Marketing/public relations specialist Copy writer/editor Web site designer Fringe benefits				
Equipment and Materials *Examples*: Office supplies Meeting supplies Computer supplies Graphic design software Data software Audio equipment Presentation equipment Other equipment purchase Computer/copier Maintenance				
Facilities *Examples*: Clinical space Space for group meetings Conference and meeting rooms				
Travel *Examples*: Staff meeting travel, lodging, and per diem Steering group travel and lodging Mileage associated with program implementation				
Other Non-Personnel Service Costs *Examples*: Conference call services Long distance services Web site service Transcription costs for focus group tapes				
Indirect/Overhead Costs				
Total Costs				

FIGURE 8–3. Generic budget planning worksheet.

5. Travel: Is there travel directly related to carrying out the project? Are there related travel expenses for other meetings or presentations in professional settings?

A generic budget planning worksheet is provided in Figure 8–3.

Identifying and Training Workers

As a program develops, adequate staff and/or volunteer training are essential for smooth implementation of interventions. Formal training should be provided for staff members who have a limited background in specific program areas such as health behavior change, evaluation, media communications, or coalition building. Special attention should also be given to basic skills such as planning, budgeting, personnel management, written and verbal communication, and cultural appropriateness. When a program involves local citizens, their training also becomes essential.[42] In the early phases, training of citizens is often skills-oriented. Other types of training may focus on leadership development or strategic planning. The training should be included as a necessary first step in the workplan, and the person(s) responsible for training should be listed in the workplan.

When addressing training needs, several key questions come to mind:

- In which areas does each staff member need training?
- Who should conduct the training?
- Do some people have unused skills that could be useful to your program?
- How best should community members be oriented and trained regarding your program?
- How can training be time efficient?

Pilot Testing the Intervention and Evaluation

Pilot testing is an important part of intervention development. A pilot test is a "mini-study" carried out with a small number of individuals (often twenty or fewer) to detect any problems with intervention and evaluation strategies.[43] Carefully examining the results of a pilot test can obviate problems before a large-scale intervention—where the stakes are higher—is undertaken. A pilot test allows you to[43, 44]

1. Refine the original hypotheses and/or research questions
2. Produce information that will help improve evaluation approaches
3. Improve curriculum materials or evaluation instruments

4. Test approaches for data imputation and analysis
5. Uncover politically sensitive issues, allowing program planners to better anticipate difficulties
6. Estimate costs for people, equipment, materials, and time
7. Ascertain the cultural appropriateness of interventions in diverse populations by inclusion in program development
8. Enhance the marketability of an intervention with senior agency administrators when a pilot test is successful

To the extent possible, a pilot test should be conducted in the same manner as that intended for the full program. In some cases, a pilot study may use qualitative methods, such as focus groups or individual interviews, that are not part of the main project. However, pilot tests can also provide an opportunity to examine the utility and appropriateness of quantitative instruments. Pilot test subjects should be similar to those who will be in your actual project. Generally, pilot test subjects should not be enrolled in your main project; therefore, it is sometimes useful to recruit pilot subjects from a separate geographic region.[43] Complete notes should be taken during the pilot test so that the project team can de-brief with all needed information.

THE ROLES OF COALITIONS, COMMUNITY ORGANIZING, AND ADVOCACY

The preceding steps and actions rarely happen in isolation; rather, solving complex health issues requires that agencies and community leaders work together effectively. Traditionally, community organizations were naturally occurring structures that brought together individuals to assess needs, organize resources to address those needs, and carry out actions to implement solutions. In recent years, public health professionals have recognized the need for community involvement in preventing disease and promoting healthy lifestyles and have attempted to capitalize on these naturally occurring strengths, capacities, and social structures to create health-promoting change. In doing so, some have created new organizations while others have attempted to work with existing organizations through collaborations or coalitions. A *coalition* is defined as a group of community members and/or organizations that join together for a common purpose.[45, 46] Some coalitions are focused on categorical issues, such as diabetes prevention or the reduction of infant mortality rates. Other coalitions form to address broader public health issues.

While community coalitions are growing in popularity, their ability to create healthful changes depends in part on the coalition's ability to move through various stages of development. There are many recent efforts to define and describe these various stages.[45–47] Most generally, in order for these groups to be effective, it is essential that they begin by developing a common vision of what they want to accomplish and a common set of skills to engage in the change process together. In addition, it is important that the individuals involved in the coalition build relationships as individuals and as representatives of their respective community organizations. As with other types of community-based health promotion programs, in order to be effective, coalitions may need to focus on a variety of developmental issues, such as developing a common set of skills and building trust, at different stages of program implementation. Wolff recently summarized the unique characteristics that contribute to the development of effective coalitions (Table 8–4).[48]

Coalitions may differ considerably in the roles and responsibilities of each member and the types of activities in which they wish to engage.[49] This can be thought of as a continuum of integration.[45, 46, 50] At one end of the continuum is the desire of agencies and individuals to work together to identify gaps in services, avoid duplication of services, and exchange information to allow for appropriate client referral. The next level of integration involves agencies maintaining their autonomy, agendas, and resources, but beginning to share these resources to work on an issue that is identified as common to all. The next level

Table 8–4. Unique Characteristics of Effective Community Coalitions

Characteristic	Description
1. Holistic and comprehensive	Allows the coalition to address issues that it deems as priorities; well-illustrated in the Ottawa Charter for Health Promotion[49]
2. Flexible and responsive	Coalitions address emerging issues and modify their strategies to fit new community needs
3. Build a sense of community	Members frequently report that they value and receive professional and personal support for their participation in the social network of the coalition
4. Build and enhance resident engagement in community life	Provides a structure for renewed civic engagement; coalition becomes a forum where multiple sectors can engage with each other
5. Provide a vehicle for community empowerment	As community coalitions solve local problems, they develop social capital, allowing residents to have an impact on multiple issues
6. Allow diversity to be valued and celebrated	As communities become increasingly diverse, coalitions provide a vehicle for bringing together diverse groups to solve common problems
7. Incubators for innovative solutions to large problems	Problem solving occurs not only at local levels, but at regional and national levels; local leaders can become national leaders

Source: adapted from Wolff.[48]

of integration involves each of the agencies lessening their level of autonomy and beginning to develop joint agendas, common goals, and shared resources.

Not all coalition efforts are successful,[51, 52] and some researchers have suggested that the impacts of coalitions have gone undetected because of inappropriate (or weak) evaluation plans. This is most likely to occur when: (1) the evaluation time line is too short; (2) the evaluation strategy focuses on unrealistic, distant health outcomes instead of intermediate indicators influenced by coalition activity; (3) measures are incapable of detecting valid indicators of change; or (4) alternative explanations for effects are not taken into account.[53] For many coalition or partnership endeavors, a realistic scaling back of expectations will offer more opportunities for accountability. Several investigators have demonstrated, for example, that it is quite feasible to establish a system to document changes in community systems and/or policies related to coalition activities.[14, 54] When these changes are documented cumulatively over time, they reflect a reasonable and appropriate reflection of a coalition's immediate impact.

The Role of Advocacy

Coalitions can have a goal of developing a program or they may be involved in more policy-level activities. In particular, community-based coalition activities may focus on advocacy. Advocacy involves a set of skills that can be employed to alter public opinion and mobilize resources in favor of a public health policy or issue.[31] The public gets much of its information about health via the media. In a 1998 national survey of adults, television was reported as the number one source for health information (39%), ranking higher than health professionals (37%).[55] Respondents also reported that the news media influenced their behavior: 35% reported that they had talked with their doctor about a medical condition as a direct result of seeing a story about it in the media, and 54% reported that they changed a health behavior (e.g., diet) because of something reported by the media.

Media advocacy has been defined as the use of media to promote a social or policy initiative.[56, 57] The goal of media advocacy is to change the way that an issue is understood by the public and by policy makers and to empower groups or individuals to take action. Although media advocacy does not directly determine health-related behaviors, it often increases a community's knowledge about a public health issue, frames the issue, and stimulates public discussion about it.[57, 58] It is therefore an important mediator of health behaviors in that it attempts to overcome structural barriers like political, economic and cultural factors that affect public health.[59] The creative use of data is very important in media advocacy. Accurate and well-known statistics can be packaged creatively so that they are interesting to the public and highlight the importance of the issue being addressed. Creative presentation of study results also enhances the interest of media professionals and provides an opportunity to communicate to the public and policymakers through editorials and news reports.

SUMMARY

This chapter provides an overview of various approaches to action planning along with several related issues. An important caveat should be kept in mind when planning an intervention. It has been suggested that sometimes a disproportionate amount of effort and resources goes into the planning process compared with the actual intervention.[60] The diagnostic phases are often resource-intensive in order to avoid action planning that leads to weak interventions. The key is to expend enough resources during the needs assessment process to be sure a problem is potentially solvable, while ensuring that adequate resources are available for later intervention approaches. It is also crucial that well-trained practitioners are available for intervention delivery.

Key points from this chapter include the following:

- Behavioral change theories are especially useful when they relate to individual-level interventions
- Ecological frameworks show promise, especially for comprehensive, multilevel interventions
- A stepwise and systematic approach to action planning can enhance the chances of program success
- Coalitions are popular vehicles for delivering population-based interventions, but realistic intermediate endpoints for coalition-based interventions should be established

SUGGESTED READINGS AND WEBSITES

Readings

Glanz K, Lewis FM, Rimer BK, eds. *Health Behavior and Health Education*. 2nd ed. San Francisco: Jossey-Bass Publishers, 1997.

McLeroy KR, Bibeau D, Steckler A, Glanz K. An ecological perspective on health promotion programs. *Health Education Quarterly* 1988;15:351–377.

Timmreck TC. *Planning, Program Development, and Evaluation. A Handbook for Health Promotion, Aging and Health Services*. Boston: Jones and Bartlett Publishers, 1995.

Green LW, Kreuter MW. *Health Promotion Planning: An Educational and Ecological Approach*. 3rd ed. Mountain View, CA: Mayfield, 1999.

Selected Websites

The Community Toolbox <http://ctb.lsi.ukans.edu/> How-to sections use simple, friendly language to explain how to do the various tasks necessary for community health and development. There are sections on leadership, strategic planning, community assessment, advocacy, grant writing, and evaluation, to give just a few examples. Each section includes a description of the task, advantages of doing it, step-by-step guidelines, examples, checklists of points to review, and training materials.

Health Education Resource Exchange (HERE) in Washington <http://www.doh.wa.gov/here/> A clearinghouse of public health education and health promotion projects, materials and resources in the state of Washington. This website is designed to help community health professionals share their experience with colleagues. The website includes sections on community projects, educational materials, health education tools, and best practices.

Healthy People 2010 Toolkit <http://www.health.gov/healthypeople/state/toolkit/> The Toolkit provides guidance, technical tools, and resources to help states, territories, and tribes develop and promote successful state-specific Healthy People 2010 plans. It can also serve as a resource for communities and other entities embarking on similar health planning endeavors.

The Planned Approach to Community Health <http://www.cdc.gov/nccdphp/patch/> The Planned Approach to Community Health (PATCH), developed by the Centers for Disease Control and Prevention and its partners, is widely recognized as an effective model for planning, conducting, and evaluating community health promotion and disease prevention programs. It is used by diverse communities in the United States and several nations to address a variety of health concerns such as cardiovascular disease, HIV, injuries, teenage pregnancy, and access to health care. The PATCH Guide is designed to be used by the local coordinator and contains "how to" information on the process, things to consider when adapting the process to a community, and sample overheads and handout materials.

REFERENCES

1. Timmreck TC. *Planning, Program Development, and Evaluation. A Handbook for Health Promotion, Aging and Health Services*. Boston: Jones and Bartlett Publishers, 1995.
2. Fawcett SB, Francisco VT, Paine-Andrews A, Schultz JA. A model memorandum of collaboration: A proposal. *Public Health Reports*. 2000;115(2–3):174–179.
3. World Health Organization. Framework for countrywide plans of action for health promotion. Paper presented at the Fifth Global Conference for Health Promotion. Health Promotion: Bridging the Equity Gap, June 5–9, 2000; Mexico.
4. Soriano FI. *Conducting Needs Assessments. A Multidisciplinary Approach*. Thousand Oaks, CA: Sage Publications, 1995.
5. Witkin BR, Altschuld JW. *Conducting and Planning Needs Assessments. A Practical Guide*. Thousand Oaks, CA: Sage Publications, 1995.
6. Glanz K. Perspectives on using theory. In: Glanz K, Lewis FM and Rimer BK, eds. *Health Behavior and Health Education*. 2nd ed. San Francisco: Jossey-Bass Publishers, 1997, pp. 441–449.

7. Sallis JF, Owen N. Ecological models. In: Glanz K, Lewis FM and Rimer BK, eds. *Health Behavior and Health Education.* 2nd ed. San Francisco: Jossey-Bass Publishers, 1997, pp. 403–424.

8. Choi KH, Yep GA, Kumekawa E. HIV prevention among Asian and Pacific Islander American men who have sex with men: A critical review of theoretical models and directions for future research. *AIDS Education and Prevention.* 1998;10(3 Suppl): 19–30.

9. Richard L, Potvin L, Kishchuk N, Prlic H, Green LW. Assessment of the integration of the ecological approach in health promotion programs. *American Journal of Health Promotion* 1996;10(4):318–328.

10. Baker EA, Brownson CA. Defining characteristics of community-based health promotion programs. *Journal of Public Health Management and Practice* 1998;4(2):1–9.

11. McLeroy KR, Bibeau D, Steckler A, Glanz K. An ecological perspective on health promotion programs. *Health Education Quarterly* 1988;15:351–377.

12. Simons-Morton DG, Simons-Morton BG, Parcel GS, Bunker JF. Influencing personal and environmental conditions for community health: A multilevel intervention model. *Family & Community Health* 1988;11(2):25–35.

13. Breslow L. Social ecological strategies for promoting healthy lifestyles. *American Journal of Health Promotion* 1996;10(4):253–257.

14. Goodman RM, Wandersman A, Chinman M, Imm P, Morrissey E. An ecological assessment of community-based interventions for prevention and health promotion: Approaches to measuring community coalitions. *American Journal of Community Psychology* 1996;24(1):33–61.

15. Prochaska JO. *Systems of Psychotherapy: A Transtheoretical Analysis.* 2nd ed. Pacific Grove, CA, 1984.

16. Prochaska JO, DiClemente CC. Stages and processes of self-change of smoking: toward an integrative model of change. *Journal of Consulting and Clinical Psychology* 1983;51(3):390–395.

17. Prochaska JO, Velicer WF. The Transtheoretical Model of health behavior change. *American Journal of Health Promotion* 1997;12(1):38–48.

18. Israel BA. Social networks and health status: linking theory, research, and practice. *Patient Counseling in Health Education* 1982;4(2):65–79.

19. Israel BA. Social networks and social support: implications for natural helper and community level interventions. *Health Education Quarterly* 1985;12(1):65–80.

20. Eng E, Young R. Lay health advisors as community change agents. *Family and Community Health.* 1992;151:24–40.

21. Brownson RC, Eriksen MP, Davis RM, Warner KE. Environmental tobacco smoke: health effects and policies to reduce exposure. *Annual Review of Public Health* 1997; 18:163–185.

22. Milio N. Priorities and strategies for promoting community-based prevention policies. *Journal of Public Health Management and Practice.* 1998;4(3):14–28.

23. Chatters LM, Levin JS, Ellison CG. Public health and health education in faith communities. *Health Education and Behavior* 1998;25(6):689–699.

24. (Entire issue devoted to desciptions of the Planned Approach to Community Health (PATCH)). *Journal of Health Education* 23(3):131–192.

25. Glanz K, Lewis FM, Rimer BK. *Health Behavior and Health Education.* 2nd ed. San Francisco: Jossey-Bass Publishers, 1997.

26. Goodman RM. Principles and tools for evaluating community-based prevention and health promotion programs. *Journal of Public Health Management and Practice* 1998;4(2):37–47.
27. Israel BA, Cumkmings KM, Dignan MB, et al. Evaluation of health education programs: current assessment and future directions. *Health Education Quarterly* 1995; 22(3):364–389.
28. Glanz K, Lewis FM, Rimer BK. Linking theory, research, and practice. In: Glanz K, Lewis FM and Rimer BK, eds. *Health Behavior and Health Education*. 2nd ed. San Francisco: Jossey-Bass Publishers, 1997, pp. 19–35.
29. Bandura A. *Social Foundations of Thought and Action: A Social Cognitive Theory*. Englewood Cliffs, NJ: Prentice Hall, 1986.
30. Abrams DB, Emmons KM, Linnan LA. Health education and behavior. The past, present, and future. In: Glanz K, Lewis FM, and Rimer BK, eds. *Health Behavior and Health Education*. 2nd ed. San Francisco: Jossey-Bass Publishers, 1997, pp. 453–478.
31. Simons-Morton BG, Greene WH, Gottlieb NH. *Introduction to Health Education and Health Promotion*. 2nd ed. Prospect Heights, IL: Waveland Press, 1995.
32. Strecher VJ, Rosenstock IM. The Health Belief Model. In: Glanz K, Lewis FM, and Rimer BK, eds. *Health Behavior and Health Education*. 2nd ed. San Francisco: Jossey-Bass Publishers, 1997, pp. 41–59.
33. Dignan MB, Carr PA. *Program Planning for Health Education and Promotion*. 2nd ed. Philadelphia: Lea & Febiger, 1992.
34. Beresford SA, Thompson B, Feng Z, Christianson A, McLerran D, Patrick DL. Seattle 5 a Day worksite program to increase fruit and vegetable consumption. *Preventive Medicine* 2001;32(3):230–238.
35. Breckon DJ, Harvey JR, Lancaster RB. *Community Health Education: Settings, Roles, and Skills for the 21st Century*. 4th ed. Rockville, MD: Aspen Publishers, 1998.
36. Green LW, Kreuter MW. *Health Promotion Planning: An Educational and Ecological Approach*. 3rd ed. Mountain View, CA: Mayfield, 1999.
37. U.S. Dept. of Health and Human Services. *Planned Approach to Community Health: Guide for the Local Coordinator*. Atlanta: Centers for Disease Control and Prevention, 1996.
38. Davis JR, Schwartz R, Wheeler F, Lancaster R. Intervention methods for chronic disease control. In: Brownson RC, Remington PL, and Davis JR, eds. *Chronic Disease Epidemiology and Control*. 2nd ed. Washington, DC: American Public Health Association, 1998, pp. 77–116.
39. Dyal WW. *Program Management. A Guide for Improving Program Decisions*. Atlanta: Centers for Disease Control and Prevention, 1990.
40. U.S. Dept. of Health and Human Services. *Developing Objectives for Health People 2010*. Washington, DC: Office of Disease Prevention and Health Promotion, 1997.
41. King JA, Morris LL, Fitz-Gibbon CT. *How to Assess Program Implementation*. Newbury Park, CA: Sage Publications, 1987.
42. Bracht N, ed. *Health Promotion at the Community Level: New Advances*. 2nd ed. Newbury Park, CA: Sage Publications, Inc, 1999.
43. McDermott RJ, Sarvela PD. *Health Education Evaluation and Measurement. A Practitioner's Perspective*. 2nd ed. New York: WCB/McGraw-Hill, 1999.

44. Borg WR, Gall MD. *Educational Research: An Introduction.* 5th ed. White Plains, NY: Longman, 1989.
45. Butterfoss FD, Goodman RM, Wandersman A. Community coalitions for prevention and health promotion. *Health Education Research* 1993;8(3):315–330.
46. Parker EA, Eng E, Laraia B, et al. Coalition building for prevention: Lessons learned from the North Carolina Community-Based Public Health Initiative. *Journal of Public Health Management and Practice* 1998;4(2):25–36.
47. Florin P, Stevenson J. Identifying training and technical assistance needs in community coalitions: A developmental approach. *Health Education Research* 1993;8: 417–432.
48. Wolff T. Community coalition building—contemporary practice and research: Introduction. *American Journal of Community Psychology* 2001;29(2):165–172; discussion, 205–111.
49. World Health Organization. Ottawa Charter for Health Promotion. Paper presented at the International Conference on Health Promotion, Ontario, Canada, November 17–21, 1986.
50. Alter C, Hage J. *Organizations Working Together: Coordination In Interorganizational Networks.* Newbury Park, CA: Sage Publications, 1992.
51. Kreuter MW, Lezin NA, Young LA. Evaluating community-based collaborative mechanisms: implications for practitioners. *Health Promotion Practice* 2000;1:49–63.
52. Roussos ST, Fawcett SB. A review of collaborative partnerships as a strategy for improving community health. *Annual Review of Public Health* 2000;21:369–402.
53. Kreuter M, Lezin N. Coalitions, consortia and partnerships. In: Last J, Breslow L, and Green LW, eds. *Encyclopedia of Public Health.* London: MacMillan Publishers Ltd, 2002 (in press).
54. Fawcett SB, Sterling TD, Paine-Andrews A, et al. *Evaluating Community Efforts to Prevent Cardiovascular Diseases.* Atlanta: Centers for Disease Control and Prevention, 1995.
55. Rodale Press. *Survey of Public Opinion Regarding Health News Coverage.* Emmaus, PA: Rodale Press, 1998.
56. Advocacy Institute. *Smoking Control Media Advocacy Guidelines.* Bethesda, MD: National Cancer Institute, 1989.
57. Wallack L, Dorfman L, Jernigan D, Themba M. *Media Advocacy and Public Health: Power for Prevention.* Newbury Park, CA: Sage, 1993.
58. Wallack L, Dorfman L. Media advocacy: A strategy for advancing policy and promoting health. *Health Education Quarterly* 1996;23(3):293–317.
59. Chapman S, Lupton D. *The Fight for Public Health. Principles and Practice of Media Advocacy.* London: BMJ Publishing Group, 1994.
60. Steckler A, Orville K, Eng E, Dawson L. Summary of a formative evaluation of PATCH. *Journal of Health Education* 1992;23(3):174–178.

9

Evaluating the Program or Policy

You see, but you do not observe.

—Sir Arthur Conan Doyle

Evaluation is an essential part of evidence-based programs and policies. It can 1) allow for midcourse corrections and changes, 2) help determine if the program or policy has been effective, and 3) provide information for planning the next program or policy. This chapter reviews some of the key issues to consider in conducting an evaluation and provides linkages to a diverse literature (within and outside public health) for those wishing to go beyond these basics.

BACKGROUND

What Is Evaluation?

Evaluation is the process of analyzing programs and policies and the context within which they occur to determine if changes need to be made in implementation and to assess the intended and unintended consequences of programs and policies; this includes, but is not limited to, determining if they are meeting their goals and objectives. According to the *Dictionary of Epidemiology*, evaluation is, "a process that attempts to determine as systematically and objectively as possible the relevance, effectiveness, and impact of activities in light of their objectives."[1] There is considerable variation in the methods used to evaluate programs and perhaps even more variation in the language used to describe each of the various evaluation techniques. There are both quantitative and qualitative evaluation methods and techniques, with the strongest approaches generally including a blending of these. While a comprehensive review of evaluation is

194

beyond the scope of any single chapter, this chapter will review some of the critical issues to consider in conducting an evaluation such as: representation of stakeholders in all aspects of the evaluation, types of evaluation, reporting back and utilizing results, and consideration of differences between program and policy evaluation.

There has been considerable discussion in the literature about the various paradigmatic approaches to both research and evaluation. A paradigm is a set of beliefs or a model that helps to guide scientific inquiry. Many of the differences in the paradigms used to guide inquiry within public health are epistemological (i.e., they reflect different perspectives on the relationship between the inquirer and what can be known) and ontological (i.e., they reflect different perspectives on the nature of reality and what can be known about it). These issues are discussed in detail elsewhere.[2-5] While a complete discussion of these issues is beyond the intent of this chapter, it is essential to recognize that the choices one makes in this regard influence the data collected, the interpretation of the data, and the utilization of evaluation results.[3, 6-8] For example, while most individuals in the field would agree that evaluation in the absence of some stakeholder involvement is not very useful, there are instances when evaluation is conducted after the program has been completed and data have already been collected. As will be discussed in more depth later in the chapter, this limits the potential for stakeholder involvement in deciding on the types of questions to ask and data to be collected. In these instances, the evaluation decisions made are influenced by program planning decisions such as those regarding timing and available data. Alternately, there are instances where the focus of the evaluation and the type of data collected are decided by the program implementers without the input of a wider group of stakeholders because of the belief that involvement of stakeholders would somehow "contaminate" the evaluation results.

Why Evaluate?

There are many reasons for public health practitioners to evaluate programs and policies. First and foremost, practitioners in the public sector must be accountable to the state legislature, local governing officials, and citizens for the use of resources. Similarly, those working in the private and nonprofit sectors must be accountable to their constituencies including those providing the funds for programs and policy initiatives. Evaluation also forms the basis for making choices when resources are limited, in part by helping to determine the costs and benefits of the various options (for more about this, see Chapter 3). Finally, evaluation is also a source of information for making midcourse corrections, improving programs and policies, and serving as the basis for deciding upon future pro-

Table 9–1. Linkages between Program Planning and Evaluation

Program Planning Activity	Evaluation Data/Sources
Goal	• Outcome data: Assess changes in morbidity, mortality, disability, quality of life —Social indicator data —Census data —National survey data
Objectives	• Impact data: Track knowledge, attitude, and behavioral/skill changes —Programmatic surveys —Qualitative data (observations, interviews, diaries, content analysis)
Action Steps	• Process data: —Records of program attendance —Survey of participant satisfaction —Observational data of environment

grams and policies. It is closely related to the program planning issues and steps described in Chapter 8 (Table 9–1).

The Role of Stakeholders

As discussed in Chapter 4, a stakeholder is anyone who is involved in program operations, is served by the program, or will use the evaluation results.[9] It is important to include representatives of all of these groups in the design of the program or policy as well as in the design, implementation, and interpretation of evaluation results. The inclusion of these lay and professional perspectives will ensure that all voices are considered in the evaluation and that all will benefit from the evaluation. For staff, inclusion in the evaluation process can provide opportunities to develop skills and abilities in evaluation design and interpretation and can ensure that changes suggested in program implementation are consistent with their work experiences. (It is critical to assure staff that program evaluation is not evaluation of personnel.[9]) In terms of program participants, inclusion in the evaluation process can increase their sense of control over the program and ensure that their previous experiences and desires are considered when changes are made in programs and policies. Administrators and program funders need to be included to ensure that evaluation activities are conducted with an understanding of where the program or policy fits within the broader organizational or agency mission and to answer questions most urgent to these groups.[9–12] Regardless of who is included, it is essential that the relationships among these stakeholders be based on mutual trust, respect, and open communication.[3, 6]

Box 9–1. A Health Funders Group: What Are We Funding?

A group of philanthropic organizations decided that they would come together to fund a health-related program. After reviewing several proposals, they decided to fund a proposal to provide home visits by nurses to sick infants and children for those families who would not otherwise be able to get these services. The group thought the program proposal would be enhanced if they worked with a group of church-based lay health advisors, and therefore required this collaboration as a condition of funding. The collaboration was considered particularly important because the proposed clients for the program had multiple nonmedical needs (such as housing and shelter, food, electricity, clothing, etc.). When the outside evaluator was called in, the first step she took was to meet with each of the ten funders and representatives of the two agencies to determine their expectations. There were twelve different perspectives on the intent of the program, ranging from decreasing infant mortality to enhancing collaboration between agencies and to providing a specific number of certain types of home visits. The evaluator presented these numerous perspectives back to the group of health funders in a meeting with agency representatives and worked with the group to narrow in on program goals and on evaluation questions that were most important, useful, and feasible to assess, given the stage of program development and agency collaboration.

Before the evaluation, begins all key stakeholders need to agree on the program goals and objectives, along with the purpose of the evaluation. Each stakeholder is likely to harbor a different opinion about the program goals and objectives and the purpose of the evaluation, and these differences must be resolved before the evaluation plan is developed and implemented[11] (Box 9–1). There are several group process techniques that can be helpful in this regard. For example, the nominal group technique, the Delphi technique, and scenario planning (see Chapter 7) all offer opportunities for individual voices to be heard while, at the same time, providing a process for prioritization.

Once these differences have been resolved, the next step is to turn stakeholder questions into an evaluation design.[8, 13] The specific roles and responsibilities of each group of stakeholders in creating the questions that guide the evaluation and in developing the methods to collect data may vary. In some evaluation designs the stakeholders may be notified as decisions are made or have minimal input into evaluation decisions.[8] There are also other evaluation designs (participatory, collaborative, or empowerment evaluation) where stakeholders are seen as equal partners in all evaluation decisions from questions asked to types of data collected and participate in analysis and interpretation of results. Some of these designs emphasize stakeholder participation as a means of ensuring that the evaluation is responsive to stakeholder needs while other designs involve stakeholders to increase the control and ownership.[2, 3, 14, 15] The role of the stakeholders will depend in part on the desires of the stakeholders and the paradigm guiding the evaluation.[3, 7, 8]

Before data collection, all stakeholders must also agree upon the extent to which the data collected will be kept confidential, not only in terms of protecting the confidentiality of participants in data collection (a nonnegotiable condition for protecting evaluation participants), but also in terms of how information will be shared within the group of stakeholders (all at once or some notified before others). The group should also reach consensus on how and when information will be communicated outside the immediate group of stakeholders and what will be shared.[8]

TYPES OF EVALUATION

There are several types of evaluation, including those related to assessment of needs and to context, process, impact, and outcome. Each type has a different purpose and is thus appropriate at different stages in the development of the program. Initial evaluation efforts should focus on the implementation of program activities, or process evaluation. Impact evaluations and outcome evaluations are only appropriate after the program has been functioning for a sufficient amount of time to see the desired changes. The exact time will depend on the nature of the program and the changes expected or anticipated. Further, each type of evaluation involves different kinds of evaluation design and data collection methods. Choices of which evaluation types to employ are based in part on the interests of the various stakeholders.

Needs Assessment and Context

A needs assessment is appropriate before the development of a program or policy, and it should answer the questions, "Is a program or policy needed to address the concern at hand?" and "What program is necessary, given a public health concern and the current resources already in place to address the concern?" Much of the data required to answer questions related to need are available through surveillance systems and national and local data sets such as those available through hospital and other service provider records, the Centers for Disease Control and Prevention (CDC) <http://www.cdc.gov>, state health departments, e.g., <http://www.health.state.mo.us/> and the census bureau <http://www.census.gov>. This information relates to current health status, rates of various risk behaviors and disease, and morbidity and mortality due to various causes. It is important to note, however, that much of this data is collected at a state or county level, making it difficult to determine the exact needs of a particular community whether it is defined as a smaller geographic area or as a nongeographic community, such as a work setting or a religious organization. There are also some data available that provide a picture of currently existing programs related to the issue or concern at hand and the population they serve <http://www.communityconnection.org/>. Other information that is useful at this stage (and through the stage of process evaluation) is documentation of the context, or setting, within which the health concern is occurring, including an assessment of the social, economic, and physical environment factors.[3, 6, 7, 9, 16] Lastly, in order to fully assess context, it is important to document the current knowledge and attitudes of potential program participants and/or those who will be affected by a program with regard to various behaviors and their perspectives on current programs (e.g., the reasons why these programs are or are not effective in meeting the defined needs).[3, 8, 9] These data can be collected through quantitative (questionnaires) or qualitative (individual or group interviews) methods.

Once these data are collected and analyzed by the identified stakeholders, a program plan must be developed. (Chapter 8 describes this process in depth.) The program plan is essential to evaluation. A key component of the program plan is the development of a logic model or a program theory (an analytic framework). A logic model lists specific activities and predicts how they will lead to the accomplishment of objectives and how these objectives will enhance the likelihood of accomplishing program goals. A logic model lays out what the program participants will do (attend an educational session on breast cancer screening at their church), what it will lead to (increased knowledge regarding risk factors for breast cancer and specific methods of breast cancer screening), which will in turn have an impact (increase breast cancer screening rates), with the intention that this will therefore produce a long term outcome (decreased morbidity due to breast cancer). While several authors have conceptualized this process somewhat differently,[7, 8, 15, 17, 18] the overall intent is that the program or policy must be laid out in such a way that it specifies the activities and the program objectives that are expected to affect clearly delineated proximal and distal outcomes. While any logic model is obviously limited in its ability to predict the often important unintended consequences of programs and policies, many argue that, even with this limitation, a logic model is mandatory to evaluate a program effectively. Rossi and colleagues have stated,[8] "evaluation in the absence of this results in a "black box" effect in that the evaluation may provide information with regard to the effects but not the processes that produced or failed to produce these effects." Moreover, because so many of the distal outcomes in health education and promotion are not evident until long after a program is implemented (e.g., decreases in morbidity due to lung cancer), it is essential to ascertain if more proximal outcomes (e.g., decreases in current smoking rates) are being achieved.

Process

Process evaluation addresses the questions of program implementation: "To what extent is the program being implemented as planned?" "Are program materials and content appropriate for the population being served?" "Who is attending educational sessions?" "Are all potential participants participating equally?" "Does the program have sufficient resources?" "What percent of the program are most participants receiving?" These data are important to document changes that have been, and need to be, made to the program to enable the program to be implemented at other sites. Information for process evaluation can be collected through quantitative and qualitative methods, including observations, field notes, interviews, questionnaires, program records, and local newspapers and publications. Box 9–2 describes a process evaluation that led to critical changes in program implementation. There are several other good examples of process evaluation.[17, 19, 20]

Impact

Impact evaluation assesses the extent to which program objectives are being met. Some also refer to this as an assessment of intermediate or proximal outcomes, both to acknowledge the importance of short-term outcomes and the fact that impact evaluation can assess intended as well as unintended consequences.[3] There are numerous useful examples of impact evaluation.[21–25]

Impact evaluation requires that all program objectives be clearly specified. A challenge in conducting an impact evaluation is the presence of many program objectives and their variable importance across stakeholders. There are also instances when a national program is implemented at many sites.[26] The national program is likely to require each site to track the attainment of certain objectives and goals. Each site, however, may also have different specific program objectives and activities that they enact to accomplish local and national objectives and achieve the desired changes in outcomes. They may, therefore, be interested in tracking these local program activities and objectives in addition to the national requirements for reporting on program outcomes. Because no evaluation can evaluate all program components, stakeholders should come to an agreement as to which objectives should be measured at what times prior to collecting data. It may be appropriate to alternate the types of data collected over months or years of a program to meet multiple programmatic and stakeholder needs. For

Box 9–2. When Outsiders Plan: Breast Cancer Screening Materials and Methods

Based on an earlier needs assessment, a program was developed to increase utilization of breast cancer screening. The program was designed to provide women over 50 with either a brochure alone or with a brochure and community outreach program in order to compare the distribution and acceptance of the information provided. After these initial program decisions were made, a program team was assembled, with individual team members ranging in age from 25 to 30 coming from four different states. As a result, none of the individuals planning the specific program strategies matched the individuals who were to receive the intervention either in terms of age or geographic region. Knowing that these differences might lead to inappropriate services, efforts were made to evaluate the materials created (an informational brochure) and methods of community outreach. A focus group was convened to review the brochure. Results indicated that the information itself was at the appropriate reading level and covered the material considered important, but was nonetheless not appropriate for the population. In an effort to make the brochure visually appealing, a speckled gray paper was used, and the ink used to print the information was a matching light gray. Women in the focus group reminded us that those with poorer eyesight, particularly older women, would have difficulty discerning the letters from the paper.

Focus groups were held to ascertain the best methods of conducting the community outreach programs. The results suggested that the format had to be enjoyable (women were tired of boring health lectures), and the intervention needed to be provided to women where they normally gathered, or at least in groups that they normally attended, rather than asking them to come to something separate from their natural social networks. Participants also noted that women would not attend sessions in buildings that had traditionally been off limits to them such as men's social clubs. The program was created to fit within these recommendations and generally had an attendance of fifteen to twenty women at each session. Some women attended more than one session because they found them enjoyable. At one site, however, there was consistently poor attendance. Participants from the focus group were asked for their insight into why there was such low attendance. They said they were not surprised at all. After all, the site chosen—a local community center—used to be an Elks Club!

example, during the initial phases of a program, it may be important to collect baseline data to meet both local and national objectives. After that point, it may be reasonable to alternate the data collected at various data collection times (time 2—data for local objectives; time 3—data for national objectives). Moreover, impact evaluation should not occur until participants have completed the program as planned or until policies have been established and implemented for some time. For example, if a program is planned to include five educational sessions, it is not useful to assess impact on objectives after the participants have attended only two sessions. It is also important to include assessments after the program has been completed to determine if the changes made as a result of the program have been sustained over time.

Program objectives assessed by impact evaluation may include changes in knowledge, attitudes, or behavior. For example, changes in knowledge about risk factors associated with breast cancer and/or the benefits of early detection might be tracked through the use of a questionnaire administered before and after an educational campaign or program. Similarly, changes in attitude might be ascertained by assessing a participant's intention to obtain a mammogram both before and after an intervention through the use of a questionnaire.

Changes associated with health promotion and disease prevention programs can be tracked through the use of pre–post questionnaires. It is often useful to use items from questionnaires that have already been used to evaluate other programs. These items are often available in peer-reviewed articles on the subject of interest (see Chapter 6 on reviewing the scientific literature). If the items are not included in the article, it is often possible to contact the researcher and obtain the items or questionnaire directly from them. In addition, programs can consider using measures that have been used in various surveillance systems such as the Behavioral Risk Factors Surveillance System, especially items on diet, physical activity, mammography, smoking. Items that have been used either in published reports or in surveillance systems are beneficial in that they have often been evaluated to ensure that the measures are both reliable and valid.

As described in more depth in Chapter 2, "validity" is the extent to which a measure accurately captures what it is intended to capture and "reliability" is the likelihood that the instrument will get the same result time after time.[27] Even if the instruments under consideration have been shown to be valid and reliable, it may be important to assess the reliability and validity of measures in the particular population being served by the program. It may be necessary to translate the items from English into other languages in a way that ensures that participants understand the meaning of the questions. This may require more than a simple word-for-word translation. In addition, the multicultural nature of public health necessitates that the methods used to collect data and the analysis and reporting of the data reflect the needs of diverse populations.[7, 28, 29] It is important to determine that the measures are appropriate for the population that is to be surveyed as is the specific program in terms of content (meeting program objectives), format (including readability), and method of administering the questionnaire (e.g., self-administered versus telephone).[30]

It is also important to consider the evaluation design that is most appropriate to assess the impact of a program or policy. While this is described in depth in Chapter 6, there are a few additional considerations, particularly when conducting community-based programs. One particularly important issue to consider is the unit of assignment to intervention or control versus unit of analysis. Braverman[31] suggests that there are many ways to address these concerns. For example, by using the individual as the unit of analysis, it is possible to use relatively fewer communities and collect more data, adjusting for the correlation among individuals within the same unit of assignment (e.g., within communities or within schools) through statistical means. Alternately, one can collect less data across more communities or separate the communities into tracks with some receiving the interventions and others being assigned to a control or delayed treatment group.[31] Others have suggested that the use of control groups may not necessarily be the best approach. Rather, the use of naturalistic inquiry and case studies, which provide in-depth descriptions of single or multiple cases, may be more useful in some evaluations.[3-5, 32-35]

Qualitative data collection, such as individual or group interviews, can also be used to evaluate program impact by documenting changes, exploring the factors related to these changes, and determining the extent to which the intervention, as opposed to other factors, has influenced these changes. Moreover, qualitative data can be particularly helpful in assessing the unintended consequences of programs and policies.[3] Qualitative data must also adhere to standards and criteria of excellence, but these criteria are different than those used for quantitative measures. Lincoln and Guba[4, 5, 36] lay out a series of expectations and criteria for ensuring rigor when using qualitative methods. These move from traditional concepts of internal validity to credibility, external validity to transferability, reliability to dependability, and objectivity to conformability. Lastly, in examining the impact of a program, some stakeholders may find it important to conduct a cost–benefit or cost–effectiveness analysis. A discussion of these methods and the advantages and disadvantages of each is provided in Chapter 3.

Outcome

Outcome evaluation provides feedback on changes in health status, morbidity, mortality, and quality of life that can be attributed to the program. These more distal outcomes are difficult to attribute to a particular program because it takes so long for the effects to be seen and because changes in these outcomes are influenced by factors outside the scope of the program itself. Assessment of a program's influence on these outcomes, therefore, is often thought to require certain types of evaluation designs (experimental and quasi-experimental rather than observational) and long-term follow-up (described in Chapter 5). Some programs, however, may rely on the published literature to extrapolate from proximal to distal outcomes. For example, the link between smoking and lung cancer is well established. Thus it may be possible to extrapolate from a decrease in smoking rates to the number of lung cancer cases prevented.

Data that are collected for purposes of outcome evaluation are more likely to be quantitative than qualitative and include social indicator data collected by state health departments, the CDC, national data sets, and local surveillance systems such as those sponsored by hospitals. Qualitative data, however, can be useful in outcome evaluations to enhance understanding of the meaning and interpretation of quantitative findings and increase credibility of the results for many stakeholders.[3]

Some kinds of data will enhance the quality of outcome evaluation. For example, it is helpful to have pre- and post-data available on the outcomes of interest. Comparison or control groups can assist in determining if the changes in desired outcomes are due to the intervention or to other factors. It is also important to have complete data; data collected as part of the program should not be systematically missing from a site or from some segment of the population of interest. In addition, secondary data, or data collected as part of surveillance systems, are most useful if they adequately and completely cover the subgroups of the population which the program or policy is intended to influence. For example, it may be important to have sufficient data to determine if there are differences in effect by race, age, or gender. The data, regardless of its source, must be collected using reliable and valid measures and be analyzed using techniques that are appropriate for the questions asked and the types of data being used.[27, 32, 33]

Indicators for Impact and Outcome Evaluation

Health indicators are measures of the extent to which targets in health programs are being reached.[37] Therefore, for purposes of evaluation, indicators are not numerical goals in themselves and should not be confused with program objectives and targets, which tend to be quantifiable according to some scale or time. Rather, indicators provide a benchmark—they can help stimulate public health action, aid program managers and policy makers in reformulating existing strategies, and assist in identifying movement toward long-term health goals. Although a large literature exists on the uses and usefulness of health indicators within medical care, much less has been published on identifying and applying indicators for impact evaluation at the community level.

Traditionally, indicators have been grouped in broad categories, focusing on sociodemographic characteristics, health status, health risk factors, health care resource consumption, functional status, and quality of life.[38] The CDC developed a consensus set of eighteen health status indicators in 1991 that are useful for outcome evaluation (Table 9–2).[39] Most of the CDC consensus indicators are measures of health status or health risk factors. They also tend to be widely available at the state, county, and city level throughout the United States. Zucconi and Carson[40] surveyed all state health departments to gain information on which of these indicators was actually being monitored. Except for work-related deaths, which were tracked in 75.5% of states, they found that mortality indicators were monitored nearly everywhere. At the county and state levels, these

Table 9–2. The Centers for Disease Control and Prevention's Consensus Set of Health Status Indicators

1. Race/ethnicity-specific infant mortality rate
2. Motor vehicle crash death rate
3. Work-related injury death rate
4. Suicide rate
5. Lung cancer death rate
6. Breast cancer death rate
7. Cardiovascular disease death rate
8. Homicide rate
9. All-cause mortality rate
10. AIDS incidence
11. Measles incidence
12. Tuberculosis incidence
13. Syphilis incidence
14. Incidence of low birth weight
15. Births to adolescents
16. Prenatal care
17. Childhood poverty
18. Proportion of persons living in counties exceeding EPA standards for air quality

Source: CDC.[39]

indicators have proven valuable in measuring progress in disease prevention and health promotion.[41] In particular, these indicators can be useful for outcome evaluation if one compares the local data with the national data and/or national goals and objectives, such as *Healthy People 2010*, and determines what might be considered realistic and achievable change within the identified community.

While adequate indicators have been developed for mortality endpoints and for many behavioral risk factors like cigarette smoking or lack of leisure-time activity, shorter-term (intermediate) markers are needed. The rationale for intermediate indicators is founded in the need for evaluators to assess program change in periods of months or years, rather than over longer periods of time. Environmental indicators (unobtrusive measures) may also be useful as an intermediate measure for documenting certain program-related changes. Examples of these indicators include the number of "No Smoking" signs or the availability of low-fat foods in local restaurants.

DECIDING ON THE APPROPRIATE EVALUATION METHODS

A review of the literature suggests that there are many issues to consider in deciding the appropriate methods to use for a particular evaluation. Several of those issues concern qualitative versus quantitative data collection. Qualitative data may include individual and group interviews; diaries of daily or weekly activities; records, newspapers and other forms of mass media; and photographs and other visual and creative arts (music, poems, etc.). Quantitative data include surveys or questionnaires, surveillance data, and other records. Either form of data may be collected as primary data (designed for purposes of the evaluation at hand) or secondary data (designed for a purpose other than the evaluation at hand, but still capable of answering the current evaluation questions to some extent).

These different types of data are often associated with different paradigmatic approaches (i.e., differences regarding what is known and how knowledge is generated) (Table 9–3). Quantitative data is generally collected using a positivist paradigm, or what is often called the "dominant" paradigm. As discussed at the beginning of this chapter, a paradigm offers guidance because it provides a set of understandings about the nature of reality and the relationship between the knower and what can be known. Within a positivist paradigm, what is known is constant, separate from the method of generating knowledge, the person conducting the inquiry, and the context within which the inquiry is conducted.[42] On the other side of the spectrum, qualitative data are often collected within alternative paradigms that include critical theory and constructionism. While these alternative paradigms vary, they generally suggest that knowledge is dependent on the context and the interaction between the researcher and the participant in a study.[42] It is important to note, however, that quantitative and qualitative data may be collected and analyzed using any paradigm as the guiding framework

Table 9–3. Comparison of Quantitative and Qualitative Evaluation Approaches

Type of Evaluation	Type of Data	Method of Collection/Analysis
Quantitative	• Survey questionnaire • Record review • Social indicator data • Geographic Information Systems • Environmental assessments	• Phone, in-person, mail • Content review • Federal (CDC WONDER, Census, BRFSS, NHANES) • Review of available data • Primary data collection, review of existing data
Qualitative	• Open-ended questions • Individual interviews • Diaries • Group interviews/focus groups • Newspapers/newsletters/printed materials • Photography • Observation/environmental assessments	• Phone, in-person, mail questionnaire • In-person, phone • Self-administered • In-person, telephone conference calls • Content analysis of archival data • Primary collection or secondary review of archival data • Single or multiple observation, structured and unstructured

for the design of the study. For example, community-based evaluations are often conducted within an alternative paradigm but may utilize either qualitative or quantitative data, or may include both types.

Using both quantitative and qualitative data is often referred to as "triangulation" of the data collection and analysis process. Triangulation generally involves the use of multiple methods of data collection and/or analysis to determine points of commonality or disagreement.[43, 44] Triangulation is often beneficial because of the complementary nature of the data. Though quantitative data provides an excellent opportunity to determine how variables are related to other variables for large numbers of people, it provides little in the way of understanding why these relationships exist. Qualitative data, on the other hand, can help provide information to explain quantitative findings, or what has been called "illuminating meaning."[44] There are many examples of the use of triangulation of qualitative and quantitative data to evaluate health programs and policies, including AIDS prevention programs,[45] occupational health programs and policies,[46, 47] and chronic disease prevention programs in community settings.[48]

Other methods of triangulation have been described. These include "investigator triangulation," in which more than one investigator collects and/or analyzes raw data.[49] When consensus emerges, the results may have higher validity. In "theory triangulation," study findings are corroborated with existing social and/ or behavioral science theories.[50]

Another important consideration in the design and implementation of the evaluation is the intent of the evaluation with regard to the creation of knowledge versus the creation of change. Many traditional forms of evaluation act to assess the extent to which a program has met its objectives. Newer methods of evaluation include participants in the evaluation process with the intent of creating changes in the social structure and increasing the capacity of participants to self-evaluate.[2] These later forms of evaluation are often called empowerment evaluation, participatory action research, or community-based participatory research.[2–4, 14, 42] Such evaluation methods assess program goals and objectives as they relate to individuals, as well as the context within which individuals live (including economic conditions, education, community capacity, social support, and control).[3, 7, 14] These approaches have been used to evaluate a variety of projects, including HIV-and AIDS-related projects, substance abuse prevention projects, and occupational health projects.[2, 51–53]

Resources, both in terms of availability and constraints, are also important to consider in determining the appropriate evaluation methods to use. Resources to consider include time, money, personnel, access to information, staff, and participants. Lastly, it is important to assess stakeholder needs in determining the type of evaluation to conduct. It may be that stakeholders require information in order to maintain program funding or to justify the program to constituents. Alternately, participants may feel that previous programs have not met their needs and may request certain types of data in order to alleviate these concerns. Similarly, program administrators in a collaborative program may require information as to the benefit of the collaboration or information on how to improve the evaluation in order to fix managerial problems that are occurring before other process, impact, or outcome measures can be assessed.

The methods of evaluation used should not, however, be constrained by the skill and comfort level of the evaluator. Because there are a broad range of evaluation skills that can be utilized and few evaluators have all of these skills, there is a temptation to see needs through the evaluator's lens of ability. It is far more useful to define the method of evaluation by the other factors mentioned above and the questions asked, and then bring together a group of evaluators who have the various skills necessary to conduct the evaluation.[3] In doing so, however, it is important to consider the ability of the evaluators to work with others who have different technical skills as well as the availability of resources to bring together these multiple types of expertise.

Policy versus Program Evaluation

While there are many similarities in using evaluation to assess the implementation and effectiveness of programs and health policy, there are some significant differences that should be noted. Just as with program planning, there are several stages in a policy cycle, including formation, design, implementation, and evaluation [11, 54–56]. In considering evaluation within the context of the policy cycle, the first decision is the utilization of evaluation in the agenda setting or policy formation stage and the policy design or formulation stage. This is similar to a needs assessment, but is likely to differ in terms of consideration of whether or not the issue warrants a public or government intervention.[11, 54–56] If there is evidence that public intervention is warranted, the question becomes whether or not current programs or legislation adequately address the concern or if there is a need to modify existing or create new programs and legislation. Issues of cost-effectiveness and public opinion are as likely to have a significant impact on the answers to these questions as other data collected.[11, 54, 56]

The next phase of the policy cycle is policy implementation.[11] Process evaluation is useful at this stage with a focus on the extent to which the policy is being implemented according to expectations of the various stakeholders. The last stage in the policy cycle is policy accountability.[11] In this stage, impact evaluation and outcome evaluation are appropriate, with a focus on the extent to which the policy has achieved its objectives and goals. These objectives include programmatic as well as structural, social, and institutional objectives and goals. For example, five years after implementation of a state law requiring insurance coverage of cancer screenings, several questions might be addressed:

• Do health-care providers know about the law?
• Do persons at risk of cancer know about the law?
• Have cancer screening rates changed?
• Are all relevant segments of the population being affected by the law?

There are several challenges in evaluating health policies. One is that the acceptable timing of the evaluation is likely to be determined more by legislative sessions than programmatic needs.[11] Because of the wide variety of objectives and goals, it is important to acknowledge from the outset that evaluation results provide but one piece of data that is used in decision making regarding maintaining or terminating a health policy. This is in part because the evaluation of public health policy must be considered part of the political process. The results of evaluations of public policy inevitably influence the distribution of power and resources. Therefore, while it is essential to conduct rigorous evaluations, it must be acknowledged that no evaluation is completely "objective," value-free, or neutral.[11, 54–56]

DISSEMINATION: REPORTING AND UTILIZING DATA

Once the data are collected and analyzed, it is important to provide the various stakeholders with a full reporting of the information collected and the recommendations for program changes. A formal report should include background information on the evaluation, such as the purpose of the evaluation (including the focus on process, impact, or outcome questions), the various stakeholders involved, a description of the program, including program goals and objectives, a description of the methodology used, and the evaluation results and recommendations.[9, 10, 16, 30, 57] Some important questions to consider when reporting evaluation data are shown in Table 9–4.[58]

Utilization of the report and the specific recommendations will depend in part on the extent to which stakeholders have been involved in the process to this point and the extent to which the various stakeholders have been involved in the data analysis and interpretation. One useful method is to conduct some sort of member validation of the findings prior to presenting a final report.[8, 9, 59] This is particularly important if the participants have not had other involvement in data analysis and interpretation. Member validation is a process by which the

Table 9–4. Questions to Consider When Reporting Evaluation Information

Question	Audience/Method for Reporting
Who are the key audiences who should be informed?	Key stakeholders (people and agencies) Participants in the program Public health practitioners Public health researchers
How will you inform the community about the results of your program?	Town meetings Meetings of local organizations (civic groups) Newspapers articles Journal articles The Internet
How can this information be used for program improvement?	Needs for new or different personnel Refinement of intervention options Changes in time lines and action steps

Source: adapted from The Planned Approach to Community Health (PATCH)[58]

preliminary results and interpretations are presented back to those who provided the evaluation data. These participants are asked to comment on the results and interpretations, and this feedback is used to modify the initial interpretations.

Utilization of the evaluation report is also influenced by its timeliness and the match between stakeholder needs and the method of reporting the evaluation results.[9, 15, 59, 60] Often, evaluation results are reported back to the funders and program administrators and published in academic journals but not provided to community-based organizations or community members themselves. The ideal method of reporting the findings to each of these groups is likely to differ. For some stakeholders, formal written reports are helpful, while for others, an oral presentation of results or information placed in newsletters or on websites might be more appropriate.[8, 10, 12] It is, therefore, essential that the evaluator considers the needs of all the stakeholders and provides the evaluation results back to the various interest groups in appropriate ways. This includes, but is not limited to, ensuring that the report enables the various stakeholders to utilize the data for future program or policy initiatives.[2, 3, 9, 14, 15, 55, 59]

SUMMARY

Evaluation is but one step in an evidence-based process of encouraging and creating health-promoting changes among individuals and within communities. As with planning, it is important to provide resources for the evaluation efforts that are appropriate to the scope of the program or policy.

Some key points from this chapter are the following:

- Because evaluation can influence the distribution of power and resources in communities, it is essential that evaluators strive to include key stakeholders from the beginning, assist program planners in clearly defining theoretically driven program goals and objectives, and seek to conduct needs assessment/ context, process, impact, and outcome evaluation as appropriate. Moreover, the information gathered must be shared with all stakeholders in ways that are understandable and useful.
- The types of data utilized (qualitative, quantitative, indicator data) must be appropriate to the questions asked. Practitioners are encouraged to seek out other experts to assist them with venturing into new data collection approaches.
- It is important to conduct an array of evaluation types (process, impact, and outcome) to ensure proper program implementation and monitoring.
- Practitioners are encouraged to publish results of their program and policy evaluations. This process creates new and sometimes generalizable knowledge that can be highly beneficial to public health professionals and, ultimately, to the communities they serve.

SUGGESTED READINGS AND WEBSITES

Readings

Fink A. *Evaluation Fundamentals: Guiding Health Programs, Research and Policy.* Newbury Park, CA: Sage Publications, 1993.

Goodman RM. Principles and tools for evaluating community-based prevention and health promotion programs. *Journal of Public Health Management and Practice* 1998; 4(2):37–47.

Israel BA, Cummings KM, Dignan MB, et al. Evaluation of health education programs: current assessment and future directions. *Health Education Quarterly* 1995;22(3):364–389.

Patton MQ. *Qualitative Evaluation and Research Methods.* Newbury Park, CA: Sage Publications, 1990.

Selected Websites

The Centers for Disease Control and Prevention Working Group on Evaluation <http://www.cdc.gov/eval/resources,htm#journals> The Centers for Disease Control and Prevention Working Group on Evaluation has developed a comprehensive list of evaluation documents, tools, and links to other websites. These materials include documents that describe principles and standards, organizations and foundations that support evaluation, a list of journals and on-line publications, and access to step-by-step manuals.

The Community Health Status Indicators (CHSI) Project <http://www.community health.hrsa.gov> The CHSI Project was launched in response to grassroots requests from local health officials for health data at the local level. The CHSI project team created 3,082 reports of health status indicators, one for each county in the nation. Secondary data were used to create these reports.

The Community Toolbox <http://ctb.lsi.ukans.edu/> These how-to sections use simple, friendly language to explain how to do the different tasks necessary for community health and development. There are sections on leadership, strategic planning, community assessment, advocacy, grant writing, and evaluation, to give just a few examples. Each section includes a description of the task, advantages of doing it, step-by-step guidelines, examples, checklists of points to review, and training materials.

The Knight Foundation <http://www.knightfdn.org> The John S. and James L. Knight Foundation website provides information on community indicators including education, well-being of children and families, housing and community development, economic development, civic engagement and positive human relations, and vitality of cultural life.

The Program Evaluation Tool Kit <http://www.uottawa.ca/academic/med/epid/toolkit.htm>This kit, available at the University of Ottawa website, provides health practitioners with an easy-to-use guide for planning and conducting small-scale process and impact evaluation. The website includes information on the tool kit as well as worksheets.

The Research Methods Knowledge Base <http://trochim.human.cornell.edu/kb/> The Research Methods Knowledge Base is a comprehensive web-based textbook that addresses all of the topics in a typical introductory undergraduate or graduate course in social research methods. It covers the entire research process, including formulating research questions; sampling (probability and nonprobability); measurement (surveys, scaling, qualitative, unobtrusive); research design (experimental and quasi-experimental); data analysis; and writing the research paper. It uses an informal, conversational style to engage both the newcomer and the more experienced research student.

REFERENCES

1. Last JM, ed. *A Dictionary of Epidemiology.* 4th ed. New York: Oxford University Press, 2001.
2. Fetterman DM, Kaftarian SJ, Wandersman A. *Empowerment Evaluation: Knowledge and Tools for Self-Assessment & Accountability.* Thousand Oaks, CA: Sage Publications, 1996.
3. Israel BA, Cumkmings KM, Dignan MB, et al. Evaluation of health education programs: Current assessment and future directions. *Health Education Quarterly* 1995; 22(3):364–389.
4. Lincoln YS, Guba EG. *Naturalistic Inquiry.* Beverly Hills, CA: Sage, 1985.
5. Lincoln YS, Guba EG. But is it rigorous? Trustworthiness and authenticity in naturalistic evaluation. In: Williams DD, ed. *Naturalistic Evaluation.* Vol 30. San Francisco: Jossey-Bass, 1986.
6. Baker EA, Homan S, Schonhoff R, Kreuter M. Principles of practice in academic-community partnerships. *American Journal of Preventive Medicine* 1999;16(3S):86–93.
7. Goodman RM. Principles and tools for evaluating community-based prevention and health promotion programs. *Journal of Public Health Management and Practice* 1998;4(2):37–47.

8. Rossi PH, Freeman HE, Lipsey MW. *Evaluation: A Systematic Approach.* 6th ed. Thousand Oaks, CA: Sage Publications, 1999.

9. Centers for Disease Control and Prevention. Framework for program evaluation in public health. *Morbidity and Mortality Weekly Report* 1999;48(RR-11):1–40.

10. Herman JL, Morris LL, Fitz-Gibbon C. *Evaluator's Handbook.* Newbury Park, CA: Sage Publications, 1987.

11. Palumbo DJ. Politics and evaluation. In: Palumbo D, ed. *The Politics of Program Evaluation.* Newbury Park, CA: Sage Publications, 1987.

12. Weiss CH. *Evaluation Research: Methods for Assessing Program Effectiveness.* Englewood Cliffs, NJ: Prentice-Hall Inc., 1972.

13. Cordray DS, Bloom HS, Light RJ. *Evaluation Practice in Review.* Vol 34. San Francisco: Jossey-Bass, 1987.

14. Parker EA, Eng E, Schulz AJ, Israel BA. Evaluating community-based health programs that seek to increase community capacity. In: Telfair J, Leviton L, and Merchant J, eds. *Evaluating Health and Human Service Programs in Community Settings.* Vol. 83. San Francisco: Jossey-Bass, 1999.

15. Patton MQ. *Utilization-focused Evaluation: The New Century Text.* 3rd ed. Thousand Oaks, CA: Sage Publications, 1997.

16. Baker QE, David DA, Gallerani R, Sanchez V, Viadro C. *An Evaluation Framework for Community Health Programs.* Durham, NC: The Center for the Advancement of Community Based Public Health, 2000.

17. Bartholomew LK, Parcel GS, Kok G. Intervention mapping: A process for developing theory and evidence based health education programs. *Health Education & Behavior.* 1998;25(5):545–563.

18. Goodman RM, Wandersman A. FORECAST: A formative approach to evaluating the CSAP comunity partnerships. *Journal of Community Psychology* 1994; CSAP special issue:6–25.

19. Stone EJ, McGraw SA, Osganian SK, Elder JP. Process evaluation in the multicenter Child and Adolescent Trial for Cardiovascular Health (CATCH). *Health Education Quarterly* 1994 ecial issue(2):S1–S148.

20. Williams JH, Belle GA, Houston C, Haire-Joshu D, Auslander WF. Process evaluation methods of a peer-delivered health promotion program for African American women. *Health Promotion Practice* 2001;2(2):135–142.

21. COMMIT Research Group. Community Intervention Trial for Smoking Cessation: Changes in adult cigarette smoking prevalence. *American Journal of Public Health* 1995;85(2):193–200.

22. COMMIT Research Group. Community Intervention Trial for Smoking Cessation: Cohort results from a four-year community intervention. *American Journal of Public Health* 1995;85(2):183–192.

23. Clark NM JN, Becker MH, Schork MA, Wheeler J, Liang J, Dodge JA, Keteyian S, Rhoads KL, Santinga JT. Impact of self-management education on the functional health status of older adults with heart disease. *Gerontologist* 1986;32:438–443.

24. COMMIT Research Group. Community Intervention Trial for Smoking Cessation: Summary of design and intervention. *Journal of the National Cancer Institute* 1991; 83:1620–1628.

25. Resnicow K, Yaroch AL, Davis A, et al. GO GIRLS! Results from a nutrition and physical activity program for low-income, overweight African American adolescent females. *Health Education of Behavior* 2000;27(5):616–632.

26. Saxe L, Tighe. The view from Main Street and the view from 40,000 feet: Can a national evaluation understand local communities? In: Telfair J, Leviton LC, and Merchant JS, eds. *Evaluating Health and Human Service Programs in Community Settings.* Vol 83. San Francisco: Jossey-Bass, 1999.
27. Kelsey JL, Petitti DB, King AC. Key methodologic concepts and issues. In: Brownson RC and Petitti DB, eds. *Applied Epidemiology: Theory to Practice.* New York: Oxford University Press, 1998, pp. 35–69.
28. Padilla AM, Medina A. Cross-cultural sensitivity in assessment using tests in culturally appropriate ways. In: Suzuki LA, ed. *Handbook of Multicultural Assessment: Clinical, Psychological and Educational Applications.* San Francisco: Jossey-Bass Publishers; 1996.
29. Suzuki LA. Multicultural Assessment: Present trends and future directions. In: Suzuki LA, ed. *Handbook of Multicultural Assessment: Clinical, Psychological, and Educational Applications.* San Francisco: Jossey-Bass Publishers, 1996.
30. Fink A. *Evaluation Fundamentals: Guiding Health Programs, Research and Policy.* Newbury Park, CA: Sage Publications, 1993.
31. Braverman MT. *Evaluating Health Promotion Programs.* Vol. 43. San Francisco: Jossey-Bass, 1989.
32. Koepsell TD, Wagner EH, Cheadle AC, et al. Selected methodological issues in evaluating community-based health promotion and disease prevention programs. *Annual Review of Public Health* 1992;13:31–57.
33. Koepsell TD. Epidemiologic issues in the design of community intervention trials. In: Brownson RC and Pettiti DB, eds. *Applied Epidemiology: Theory to Practice.* New York: Oxford University Press, 1998, pp. 177–211.
34. Balbach ED. *Using Case Studies To Do Program Evaluation.* Sacramento, CA: California Department of Health Services, 1999.
35. Yin RK. *Case Study Research: Design and Methods.* Beverly Hills, CA: Sage Publications, 1994.
36. Guba EG, Lincoln YS. The countenances of fourth-generation evaluation: Description, judgment, and negotiation. In: Palumbo D, ed. *The Politics of Program Evaluation.* Newbury Park, CA: Sage Publications, 1987.
37. World Health Organization. *Health Program Evaluation. Guiding Principles for Its Application in the Managerial Process for National Development.* Health for All Series, No.6. Geneva: World Health Organization; 1981.
38. Durch JS, Bailey LA, Stoto MA, eds. *Improving Health in the Community: A Role of Performance Monitoring.* Washington, DC: National Academy Press, 1997.
39. Centers for Disease Control. Consensus set of health status indicators for the general assessment of community health status—United States. *Morbidity and Mortality Weekly Report* 1991;40:449–451.
40. Zucconi SL, Carson CA. CDC's Consensus Set of Health Status Indicators: Monitoring and prioritization by state health departments. *American Journal of Public Health* 1994;84:1644–1646.
41. Sutocky JW, Dumbauld S, Abbott GB. Year 2000 health status indicators: A profile of California. *Public Health Reports* 1996;111:521–526.
42. Israel BA, Schulz AJ, Parker EA, Becker AB. Community-based research: A partnership approach to improve public health. *Annual Review of Public Health* 1998; 19:173–202.
43. Denzin NK. *The Research Act in Sociology.* London: Butterworth, 1970.

44. Steckler A, McLeroy KR, Goodman RM, Bird ST, McCormick L. Toward integrating qualitative and quantitative methods: An introduction. *Health Education Quarterly* 1992;19(1):1–9.
45. Dorfman LE, Derish PA, Cohen JB. Hey Girlfriend: An evaluation of AIDS prevention among women in the sex industry. *Health Education Quarterly* 1992;19(1):25–40.
46. Gottlieb NH, Lovato CY, Weinstein R, Green LW, Eriksen MP. The implementation of restrictive worksite smoking policy in a large decentralized organization. *Health Education Quarterly* 1992;19(1):77–100.
47. Hugentobler M, Israel BA, Schurman SJ. An action research approach to workplace health: Integrating methods. *Health Education Quarterly* 1992;19(1):55–76.
48. Goodman RM, Wheeler FC, Lee PR. Evaluation of the heart to heart project: Lessons from a community-based chronic disease prevention project. *American Journal of Health Promotion* 1995;9(6):443–455.
49. Guyatt G, Rennie D, eds. *Users' Guides to the Medical Literature. A Manual for Evidence-Based Clinical Practice*. Chicago: American Medical Association Press, 2002.
50. Denzin NK. *Sociological Methods*. New York: McGraw Hill, 1978.
51. Baker E, Israel B, Schurman SJ. A participatory approach to worksite health promotion. *The Journal of Ambulatory Care Management* 1994;17(2):68–80.
52. Israel BA, Schurman SJ, House JS. Action research on occupational stress: Involving workers as researchers. *International Journal of Health Services* 1989; 19(No. 1): 135–155.
53. Israel B, Schurman S, Hugentobler M, House J, eds. *A participatory action research approach to reducing occupational stress: Phases of implementation and evaluation*. DiMartino V, ed. Conditions of Work Digest: Anti-Stress Programs. Geneva: International Labor Office, 1992.
54. Chelimsky E. Linking program evaluation to user needs. In: Palumbo DJ, ed. *The Politics of Program Evaluation*. Newbury Park, CA: Sage Publications, 1987.
55. Chelimsky E. The politics of program evaluation. In: Cordray DS, Bloom HS, and Light RJ, eds. *Evaluation Practice in Review*. Vol. 34. San Francisco: Jossey-Bass, 1987.
56. Weiss CH. Where politics and evaluation reserach meet. In: Palumbo DJ, ed. *The Politics of Program Evaluation*. Newbury Park, CA: Sage Publications, 1987.
57. Morris LL, Fitz-Bibbon CT, Freeman ME. *How to Communicate Evaluation Findings*. Newbury Park, CA: Sage Publications, 1987.
58. US Department of Health and Human Services. *Planned Approach to Community Health: Guide for the Local Coordinator*. Atlanta: Centers for Disease Control and Prevention, 1996.
59. Patton MQ. *Qualitative Evaluation and Research Methods*. Newbury Park, CA: Sage Publications, 1990.
60. Patton MQ. Integrating evaluation into a program for increased utility and cost-effectiveness. In: McLaughlin JA, Weber LJ, Covert RW, and Ingle RB, eds. *Evaluation Utilization*. Vol. 39. San Francisco: Jossey-Bass, 1988.

Glossary

Action planning: Planning for a specific program or policy with specific, time-dependent outcomes.

Adjusted rates: A rate in which the crude (unadjusted) rate has been standardized to some external reference population (e.g., an age-adjusted rate of lung cancer). An adjusted rate is often useful when comparing rates over time or for populations in different geographic areas.

Advocacy: A set of skills that can be used to create a shift in public opinion and mobilize the necessary resources and forces to support an issue. Advocacy blends science and politics in a social-justice value orientation with the goal of making the system work better, particularly for individuals and populations with the least resources.

Analytic epidemiology: Study designed to examine associations, commonly putative or hypothesized causal relationships. An analytic study is usually concerned with identifying or measuring the effects of risk factors or is concerned with the health effects of specific exposures.

Analytic framework: (causal framework/logic model) A diagram that depicts the interrelationships between population characteristics, intervention components, shorter-term intervention outcomes, and longer-term public health outcomes. Its purpose is to map out the linkages on which to base conclusions about intervention effectiveness. Similar frameworks are also used in program planning to assist in designing, implementing, and evaluating effective interventions.

Basic Priority Rating (BPR): A method of prioritizing health issues based on the size of the problem, the seriousness of the problem, the effectiveness of intervention, and its propriety, economics, acceptability, resources, and legality (known as PEARL). First developed by Hanlon and Pickett.

Case-control study: The method of study in which persons with the disease (or other outcome) of interest are compared with a suitable control group of persons without the

217

disease. The relationship of an attribute to the disease is examined by comparing the diseased and nondiseased with regard to how frequently the attribute is present. Risk is estimated by the odds ratio.

Causality: The relationship of causes to the effects they produce. A cause is termed "necessary" when it must always precede an effect. This effect need not be the sole result of the one cause. A cause is termed "sufficient" when it inevitably initiates or produces an effect. Any given causal factor may be necessary, sufficient, neither, or both.

Causal framework: (logic model/analytic framework) A diagram that depicts the inter-relationships between population characteristics, intervention components, shorter-term intervention outcomes, and longer-term public health outcomes. The purpose is to map out the linkages on which to base conclusions about intervention effectiveness.

Changeability: The likelihood that a risk factor or behavior can be altered by a public health program or policy.

Clinical guideline: A systematically developed statement designed to assist clinician and patient decisions about appropriate health care for specific clinical circumstances.

Coalition: A group of individuals and/or organizations that join together for a common purpose.

Cohort study: The method of study in which subsets of a defined population can be identified by who are, have been, or in the future may be exposed or not exposed, or exposed in different degrees, to a factor or factors hypothesized to influence the proba-bility of occurrence of a given disease or other outcome. The main feature of cohort study is observation of large numbers over a long period (commonly years) with com-parison of incidence rates in groups that differ in exposure levels. Risk is estimated by the relative risk.

Community: A group of people with diverse characteristics who are linked by social ties, share common perspectives, and engage in joint action in geographical locations or settings.

Confounding: A bias that distorts the estimated effect of an exposure on an outcome, caused by the presence of an extraneous factor associated with both the exposure and the outcome

Consensus conferences: A mechanism commonly used to review epidemiologic evi-dence. Expert panels convene to develop recommendations, usually within a two and one-half day conference.

Context or Setting: The surroundings within which a health issue occurs, including assessment of the social, economic, political, and physical environment.

Cost–benefit analysis: An economic analysis that converts effects into the same monetary terms as the costs and compares them.

Cost-effectiveness analysis: An economic analysis in which the total costs of an inter-vention are measured in monetary terms and then compared with the outcomes (such as lives saved or quality-adjusted-life-years produced) achieved by the intervention.

Cost-minimization analysis: Compares the costs of different programs with equivalent benefits and bases the decision solely on cost. Generally the easiest method to use for economic evaluation yet is useful for a relatively small number of issues (e.g., comparison of generic vs. name brand drugs).

Cost-utility analysis: An economic analysis that converts effects into personal preferences (or utilities) and describes how much it costs for some additional quality gain, such as cost per additional quality-adjusted life-year. Cost-utility analysis is sometimes considered a subset of cost-effectiveness analysis.

Cross-sectional studies: The method of study in which the presence or absence of a disease and the presence or absence of other variables are determined in each member of the study population or in a representative sample at one particular time.

Decision analysis: A technique used under conditions of uncertainty for systematically representing and examining all the relevant information for a decision and the uncertainty around that information. The available choices are plotted on a decision tree. At each branch, or decision node, the probabilities of each outcome that can be predicted are estimated. The relative worth or preferences of decision makers for the various possible outcomes for a decision can also be estimated and incorporated into a decision analysis.

Delphi method: Iterative circulation to a panel of experts of questions and responses that are progressively refined in light of responses to each round of questions; preferably, participants' identities should not be revealed to each other. The aim is to reduce the number of viable options or solutions, perhaps to arrive at a consensus judgment on an issue or problem, or a set of issues or problems, without allowing anyone to dominate the process. The method was originally developed at the RAND Corporation.

Descriptive epidemiology: Study of the occurrence of disease or other health-related characteristics in human populations. General observations are often made concerning the relationship of disease to basic characteristics such as age, sex, race, social class, geographic location, or time. The major characteristics in descriptive epidemiology can be classified under the headings of person, place, and time.

Direct costs: Include labor costs, often measured by the number of full-time equivalent employees (FTEs) and their wages and fringe benefits. Direct costs also include supplies and overhead.

Dissemination: The process of communicating either the procedures or the lessons learned from a study or program evaluation to relevant audiences in a timely, unbiased, and consistent fashion.

Distal outcomes: Long-term changes in health status, morbidity, mortality, and quality of life.

Ecological framework: A model that suggests that it is important to address individual, interpersonal, organizational, community (including social and economic factors), and health policy factors because of the effect these factors have on individual behavior change and because of their direct effect on health.

Economic evaluation: Evaluations that include costs and benefits in quantitative terms. Comparison of the relationship between costs and outcomes of alternative health care interventions.

Evaluation: A process that attempts to systematically and objectively determine the relevance, effectiveness, and impact of activities in the light of their objectives.

Evaluation designs: The qualitative and quantitative methods used to evaluate a program that may include both experimental and quasi-experimental studies.

Evidence-based medicine: The conscientious, explicit, and judicious use of current best evidence in making decisions about the care of individual patients. The practice of evidence-based medicine means integrating individual clinical expertise with the best available external clinical evidence from systematic research.

Evidence-based public health: The development, implementation, and evaluation of effective programs and policies in public health through application of principles of scientific reasoning, including systematic uses of data and information systems and appropriate use of behavioral science theory and program planning models.

Experimental study design: A study in which the investigator has full control over the allocations and/or timing of the interventions. The ability to allocate individuals or groups randomly is a common requirement of an experimental study.

Expert panel: Provides scientific peer review of the quality of the science and scientific interpretations that underlie public health recommendations, regulations, and policy decisions.

External validity: A study is externally valid, or generalizable, if it can produce unbiased inferences regarding a target population (beyond the subjects in the study). This aspect of validity is only meaningful with regard to a specified external target population.

"Fugitive" literature: Government reports, book chapters, the proceedings of conferences, and published dissertations are called "fugitive" literature when the documents or their contents are difficult to retrieve. Studies published in conference proceedings, as book chapters, and in government reports are not identified in searches of MEDLINE and most other computer databases.

Guide to Clinical Preventive Services: A guideline, published by the U.S. Preventive Services Task Force, that documents the effectiveness of a variety of clinic-based interventions in public health through systematic review and evaluation of scientific evidence.

Guide to Community Preventive Services: Systematic Reviews and Evidence-Based Recommendations: A guideline, published by the Task Force on Community Preventive Services and supported by the Centers for Disease Control and Prevention (CDC) that summarizes what is known about the effectiveness and cost-effectiveness of population-based interventions designed to promote health and prevent disease, injury, disability, and premature death, as well as reduce exposure to environmental hazards.

Guidelines: A standardized set of information describing the best practices for addressing health problems commonly encountered in public health practice. Information is based on scientific evidence of the effectiveness and efficiency of the practices described. Where such evidence is lacking, guidelines are sometimes based on the consensus opinions of public health experts.

Health Belief Model: A value expectancy theory. The theory states that individuals will take action to ward off, screen for, or control an ill-health condition if they regard themselves as susceptible to the condition, believe it to have potentially serious consequences, believe that a course of action available to them would be beneficial in reducing either their susceptibility to or the severity of the condition, and believe that the anticipated barriers to (or costs of) taking the action are outweighed by its benefits.

Health indicator: A variable, susceptible to direct measurement, that reflects the state of health of persons in a community. Examples include infant mortality rates, incidence rates based on notifiable cases of disease, or disability days.

Impact evaluation: This type of evaluation assesses whether intermediate objectives have been achieved. Indicators may include changes in knowledge, attitudes, or risk-factor prevalence.

Indirect costs: There are five components including:
1. Time and travel costs to participants
2. Averted treatment costs or future treatment costs that will be saved as a result of the intervention
3. Cost of treating side effects
4. Averted productivity losses or savings to society from avoiding lost work time
5. Cost of treatment during gained life expectancy

Information bias: A bias in measuring exposures or outcomes that affects the accuracy of information between study groups.

Internal validity: The degree to which the inference drawn from a study is warranted when account is taken of the study methods, the representativeness of the study sample, and the nature of the population from which it is drawn. Index and comparison groups are selected and compared in such a manner that the observed differences between them on the dependent variables under study may, apart from sampling error, be attributed only to the hypothesized effect under investigation.

Logic model: A diagram that illustrates the sequencing of program activities that should occur for planning, organizing, implementing, and producing desired results.

Management: The process of constructing, implementing, and evaluating organized responses to a health problem or a series of interrelated health problems.

MATCH: The Multilevel Approach to Community Health is both a conceptual and practical intervention planning model. MATCH consists of five phases, including health goals selection, intervention planning, development, implementation, and evaluation.

Media advocacy: Advocacy that involves strategic use of the mass media in reaching policy, program, or educational goals.

Member validation: A process by which the preliminary results and interpretations are presented back to those who provided the evaluation data.

Meta-analysis: A systematic, quantitative method for combining information from multiple studies in order to derive the most meaningful answer to a specific question.

Multiple linear regression: Given data on a dependent variable y and several independent variables x_1, x_2, etc., regression analysis involves finding the "best" mathematical model to describe y as a function of the x's according to a linear model. Other common regression models in epidemiology are the logistic and proportional hazards models.

Needs assessment: A systematic procedure for determining the nature and extent of problems experienced by a specified population that affect their health either directly or indirectly. Needs assessment makes use of epidemiologic, sociodemographic, and qualitative methods to describe health problems and their environmental, social, economic, and behavioral determinants. The aim is to identify unmet health care needs and preventive opportunities.

Nominal Group Technique: A structured, small group process that involves in-person interactions in the same room. Generally six to ten members represent a group in name only, and may not always interact as a group in a typical work setting. The nominal group technique can be useful in generating creative and innovative alternatives and is more feasible for routine decisions.

Objectivity: The ability to be unaffected by personal biases, politics, history, or other external factors.

Observational study design: A study that does not involve any intervention, experimental or otherwise. Such a study may be one in which nature is allowed to take its course, with changes in one characteristic being studied in relation to development of disease or other health condition. Examples of observational studies include the cohort study or the case-control study.

Odds ratio: The ratio of the odds of an event in the exposed group to the odds of an event in the control (unexposed) group. Commonly used in the case-control method to estimate the relative risk. The prevalence odds ratio is often calculated for cross-sectional data.

Original research articles: A paper written by the author(s) who conducted the research.

Outcome evaluation: The long-term measures of effects such as changes in morbidity, mortality, and quality of life.

Paradigm: A typical example, a pattern of thought or conceptualization, an overall way of regarding phenomena within which scientists normally work.

PATCH (The Planned Approach to Community Health): A community health planning model that relies heavily on local data to set priorities, design interventions, and evaluate progress. The goal of PATCH is to increase the capacity of communities to plan, implement, and evaluate comprehensive, community-based interventions.

Peer review: Process of reviewing research proposals, manuscripts submitted for publication, and abstracts submitted for presentation at scientific meetings, whereby they are judged for scientific and technical merit by other scientists in the same field.

PERT: (Program Evaluation and Review Technique): A graphically displayed time line for the tasks necessary in the development and implementation of public health programs.

Policy: Laws, regulations, and formal and informal rules and understandings that are adopted on a collective basis to guide individual and collective behavior.

Population attributable risk (PAR): The incidence of a disease in a population that is associated with or attributable to exposure to the risk factor.

Population-based process: An administrative strategy that seeks to maximize expected health and well-being across an entire community or population, rather than maximizing outputs and outcomes within specific programs and organizations.

PRECEDE-PROCEED: A systematic planning framework developed to enhance the quality of health education interventions. The acronym PRECEDE stands for Predisposing, Reinforcing, and Enabling Constructs in Educational Diagnosis and Evaluation. The model is based on the premise that, just as medical diagnosis precedes a treatment plan, so should educational diagnosis precede an intervention plan. The acronym PROCEED stands for Policy, Regulatory, and Organizational Constructs in Educational and Environmental Development. This part of the model is based on recognition of the need for health promotion interventions that go beyond traditional educational approaches to changing unhealthy behaviors.

Precision: The quality of being sharply defined or stated. In statistics, precision is defined as the inverse of the variance of a measurement or estimate.

Preventable burden (preventability; prevented fraction): The proportion of an adverse health outcome that potentially can be eliminated as a result of a prevention strategy.

Preventability: The potential effects of the intervention.

Process evaluation: The analysis of inputs and implementation experiences to track changes as a result of program or policy. This occurs at the earliest stages of public health intervention and often is helpful in determining midcourse corrections.

Program: An organized public health action, including direct service interventions, community mobilization efforts, policy development and implementation, outbreak investigations, health communication campaigns, health promotion programs, and applied research initiatives.

Program objectives: Statements of short-term, measurable, specific activities having a specific time limit or timeline for completion. Program objectives must be measurable and are used to reach goals.

Public health surveillance: The ongoing collection and timely analysis, interpretation, and communication of health information for public health actions.

Publication bias: A bias in the published literature where the publication of research depends on the nature and direction of the study results. Studies in which an intervention is not found to be effective are sometimes not published or submitted for publication. Therefore, systematic reviews that fail to include unpublished studies may overestimate the true effect of an intervention or risk factor.

Quality-adjusted life-years (QALYs): A frequently used outcome measure in cost-utility analysis that incorporates the quality of desirability of a health state with the duration of survival. The quality of life is integrated with the length of life by using a multiplicative formula.

Quality of the evidence: Quality refers to the appropriateness and integrity of the information obtained. High-quality data are reliable, valid, and informative for their intended use.

Qualitative data: Nonnumerical observations, using approved methods such as participant observation, group interviews, or focus groups. Qualitative data can enrich understanding of complex problems and help to explain why things happen.

Quantitative data: Data in numerical quantities, such as continuous measurements or counts.

Quasi-experimental designs: A study in which the investigator lacks full control over the allocation and/or timing of intervention but nonetheless conducts the study as if it were an experiment, allocating subjects to groups. Inability to allocate subjects randomly is a common situation that may be best studied as a quasi-experiment.

Randomized controlled trials: An experiment in which subjects in a population are randomly allocated into groups, usually called study and control groups, to receive or not to receive an experimental preventive or therapeutic procedure, maneuver, or intervention.

Rate: A rate is a measure of the frequency of occurrence of a phenomenon (e.g. a disease or risk factor) for a defined population during a specified period.

Registries: Listings maintained and updated of individuals with specific diseases or health problems. Active registries seek data and use follow-up to obtain more reliable and complete information. Passive registries accept and merge reports but do not update or confirm information.

Relative risk: The ratio of the rate of disease or death among the exposed to the rate among the unexposed; synonymous with rate ratio or risk ratio.

Relative standard error: A standard error (i.e. the standard deviation of an estimate) as a percentage of the measure itself. A relative standard error of 50% means the standard error is half the size of the rate. For crude mortality and incidence rates, the relative standard error is equal to:

$$\frac{1}{\sqrt{no. \ of \ cases}}*100$$

Reliability: The degree of stability exhibited when a measurement is repeated under identical conditions. Reliability refers to the degree to which the results obtained by a measurement procedure can be replicated. Lack of reliability may arise from divergences between observers or instruments or instability of the attribute being measured.

Reportable diseases: Mandated by law and/or regulation at national, state, and local levels, data are collected on selected diseases.

Resource-based decision making: In the resource-based planning cycle, the spiral of increased resources and increased demand for resources helps to drive the cost of health care services continually higher, even as the health status for some populations decline.

Review articles: A summary of what is known on a particular topic through review of original research articles.

Risk assessment: The qualitative and quantitative estimation of the likelihood of adverse effects that may result from exposure to specified health hazards or from the absence of beneficial influences.

Scenario planning: In this small group method, future-oriented scenarios are developed, based on how and event or system will look at some target time horizon. In some cases, scenario planning has been used when other, more quantitative, forecasting methods fail to anticipate a changing environment.

Scientific literature: Refers to theoretical and research publications in scientific journals, reference books, textbooks, government reports, policy statements, and other materials about the theory, practice, and results of scientific inquiry.

Selection bias: A bias (error) due to systematic differences in characteristics between those who take part in the study and those who do not.

Sensitivity analysis: An analysis used to determine how sensitive the results of a study or systematic review are to changes in how it was done. Sensitivity analyses are used to assess how robust the results are to uncertain decisions or assumptions about the data and the methods that were used.

Small area analyses: As a rough guide, a small area is defined as one containing fewer than twenty cases of the disease of interest. Because small area analyses tend to deal with low incidence events, special considerations and statistical tests may be necessary to deal with small numbers.

Stakeholder: An individual or organization with an interest in an intervention, health policy, or health outcome.

Strategic planning: Detailed plans including objectives and a set of essential actions (preventive and therapeutic) believed sufficient to control a health problem.

Survey: An investigation in which information is systematically collected but in which the experimental method is not used. The information collected almost always needs editing, coding, data entry, and data analysis. Survey data differ from surveillance data in that they are not on-going but rather sporadic.

SWOT analysis: A SWOT analysis (identification of the internal Strengths and Weaknesses of the organization, and external Opportunities and Threats that face the organization) brings the resources and gaps (strengths and weaknesses) within the organization into focus while looking at the impact of external forces (opportunities and threats).

Systematic review: A review of a clearly formulated question that uses systematic and explicit methods to identify, select, and critically appraise relevant research, and to collect and analyze data from the studies that are included in the review. Statistical methods (meta-analysis) may or may not be used to analyze and summarize the results of the included studies.

Time-series analyses: A quasi-experimental research design in which measurements are made at several different times, thereby allowing trends to be detected.

Triangulation: Triangulation generally involves the use of multiple methods of data collection and/or analysis to determine points of commonality or disagreement. It often involves a combination of qualitative and quantitative data.

Transferability: The degree to which the results of a study or systematic review can be extrapolated to other circumstances, in particular to routine health care situations.

Transtheoretical model: A theory of health behavior change. It suggests that people move through one of five stages and that health behavior change is an evolving process that can be more effectively achieved if the intervention of choice matches the stage of readiness to change behavior.

Type I evidence: Analytic data showing the importance of a particular health condition and its link with some preventable risk factor. For example, a large body of epidemiologic evidence shows that smoking causes lung cancer.

Type II evidence: Data that focuses on the relative effectiveness of specific interventions to address a particular health condition. For example, a growing body of evidence shows that several interventions are effective in preventing the uptake (initiation) of smoking in youth.

Unit of analysis: The unit of assignment in an intervention study. Most commonly, the unit will be an individual person but, in some studies, people will be assigned in groups to one or another of the interventions. This is done either to avoid contamination or for convenience, and the units might be schools, hospitals, or communities.

Vital statistics: Information compiled by state health agencies concerning births, deaths, marriages, divorces, and abortions.

REFERENCES

Some definitions are adapted from the following sources:

Brownson RC, Gurney JG, Land G. Evidence-based decision making in public health. *Journal of Public Health Management and Practice* 1999;5:86–97.

Centers for Disease Control and Prevention. Framework for program evaluation in public health. *Morbidity and Mortality Weekly Report* 1999;48(RR-11):1–40.

Cuzick J, Elliott P. Small area studies: Purpose and methods. In: Elliott P, Cuzick J, English D, and Stern R, eds. *Geographical and Environmental Epidemiology: Methods for Small Area Studies.* Oxford: Oxford University Press, 1992, pp. 14–21.

Ginter PM, Swayne LM, Duncan WJ. *Strategic Management of Health Care Organizations.* 3rd ed. Malden, MA: Blackwell Publishers Inc., 1998.

Glanz K, Lewis FM, Rimer BK, eds. *Health Behavior and Health Education.* 2nd ed. San Francisco: Jossey-Bass Publishers, 1997.

Goodman RM. Principles and tools for evaluating community-based prevention and health promotion programs. *Journal of Public Health Management and Practice* 1998; 4(2):37–47.

Green LW. Health education's contribution to public health in the twentieth century: A glimpse through health promotion's rear-view mirror. *Annual Review of Public Health* 1999;20:67–88.

Haddix AC, Teutsch SM, Shaffer PA, Dunet DO, eds. *Prevention Effectiveness. A Guide to Decision Analysis and Economic Evaluation.* New York: Oxford University Press, 1996.

Hanlon J, Pickett G. *Public Health Administration and Practice.* Santa Clara, CA: Times Mirror/Mosby College Publishing; 1982.

Last JM, ed. *A Dictionary of Epidemiology*, 4th Edition ed. New York: Oxford University Press, 2001.

MacQueen KM, McLellan E, Metzger DS, et al. What is community? An evidence-based definition for participatory public health. *American Journal of Public Health* 2001; 91(12):1929–1938.

Novick LF, Mays GP, eds. *Public Health Administration Principles for Population-Based Management.* Gaithersburg, MD: Aspen, Inc., 2001.

Sackett DL, Straus SE, Richardson WS, Rosenberg W, Haynes RB. *Evidence-Based Medicine. How to Practice and Teach EBM.* 2nd ed. Edinburgh: Churchill Livingston, 2000.

Schmid TL, Pratt M, Howze E. Policy as intervention: Environmental and policy approaches to the prevention of cardiovascular disease. *American Journal of Public Health* 1995;85(9):1207–1211.

Simons-Morton BG, Greene WH, Gottlieb NH. *Introduction to Health Education and Health Promotion.* 2nd ed. Prospect Heights, IL: Waveland Press, 1995.

Wallack L, Dorfman L, Jernigan D, Themba M. *Media Advocacy and Public Health: Power for Prevention.* Newbury Park, CA: Sage, 1993.

Witkin BR, Altschuld JW. *Conducting and Planning Needs Assessments. A Practical Guide.* Thousand Oaks, CA: Sage Publications, 1995.

Index